Dear Raven and Joshua

Questions and Answers About
Master/Slave Relationships

Raven Kaldera and Joshua Tenpenny

DEAR RAVEN AND JOSHUA
Questions and Answers About
Master/Slave Relationships

Raven Kaldera and Joshua Tenpenny

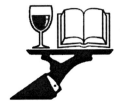

Alfred Press
Hubbardston, Massachusetts

Alfred Press
12 Simond Hill Road
Hubbardston, MA 01452

Dear Raven and Joshua: Questions and Answers
About Master/Slave Relationships
© 2009 Raven Kaldera and Joshua Tenpenny
ISBN 978-0-578-03460-7

Front cover photo by Corwin Samuelson.
Back cover photo by Sensuous Sadie.

Printed in cooperation with
Lulu Enterprises, Inc.
860 Aviation Parkway, Suite 300
Morrisville, NC 27560

Dedicated to our family,
who put up with us.

Contents

Introduction

The world of consensual Master and slave relationships is usually seen as a shadowed and nebulous land, full of dark corners and obscure dangers. It is usually viewed from afar through a haze of sexual fantasy, and usually goes no further than that. Couples who venture in with the fantasy-glasses often find all too quickly that it wasn't what they thought it would be, and wander off to new fantasy fields, proclaiming that such things "don't really happen in real life". The few who stay and struggle their way to a deeper truth, one not ruled by the libido, often stay silent on the topic of their mistakes in getting to that place, and staying there.

We found ourselves in this place, eight years prior to this day as we add the last finishing touches to this manuscript. Raven wanted a slave boy and Joshua wanted to be that slave boy, and we jumped the cliff with little preparation or idea where to go. Most of the information we found, we scrapped as being too unrealistic, and we did it alone through trial and error. We were sure of a few things: that Raven was naturally dominant in relationships and that Joshua was naturally submissive; that whenever we came together we fell almost automatically into those roles, to the point where it was painful to be any other way; that we both saw the giving and receiving of service and mastery as part of a spiritual path. Anything else, we could figure out on our own.

Over the years, we began to speak about our relationship and people began to ask us questions ... and by that time we'd both collected long lists of fallacies about M/s relationships that were still being perpetuated. We began not only to speak but to speak out, and to write down our answers, some of which we ended up saying over and over.

This is a book of those questions. Versions of some of those questions were brought up to us by people who slipped by after we gave workshops and presentations on M/s and asked questions with worried looks on their faces. Versions of others were emailed to us personally by troubled couples trying to do this work without any role models, and still others were addressed to a large group of people on various online forums that discussed Master/slave and Dominant/submissive relationships. Some were unusual and memorable enough that we decided to include them, after rewriting them for clarity and significantly changing the wording to apply to a greater audience. Others were asked so many times by so many different people that we created versions that were composites of the original problems. In no case did we use a question with its original wording.

Some of the questions are answered by both of us, some by one or the other as we were inspired or had specific knowledge. Sometimes—what a shock!—we even disagree. Well, a little, anyway. Our power dynamic does not require that Joshua agree with everything that Raven says— obedience does not mean brainlessness—and for the sake of honesty we included differing replies in this book.

These questions and answers don't cover everything that anyone could possibly learn about Master/slave relationships; in fact, there will probably be huge gaps in the information. (For example, there's a lot of important material that we didn't put in regarding spirituality, partly because the book was already too long and partly because we'd covered so much of that in Raven's book, *Dark Moon Rising*.) These relationships are a far more complex subject than people might believe. Anything to do with human relationships is complicated, and unusual relationship structures add an extra layer of complication. These questions are just the "top hundred" that we get asked on a regular basis. Our answers are opinionated, so if you don't agree with any one of them, feel free to skip it.

By no means is our M/s relationship perfect. It's a work in progress, just like everything else we do. We make mistakes, we backslide on rules and have to discipline ourselves, we let stress and illness disrupt the free flow of our dynamic, we get angry and frustrated ... but after all this time, we have a variety of tools to pull ourselves together and get back on track. Don't think, as you read, that we are infallible. We've just managed to amass some useful skills, which we hope to pass on here. (And the day that we have the hubris to decide that we've got it all down perfectly, the Universe will probably arrange for us to have a nice big public fight in the hotel lobby of a kink conference where we're about to speak on how to do a M/s relationship properly. To be mindful is to be humble.)

We are part of a minority within a minority within a minority. Of the demographic of people who are attached in any way to BDSM communities, the majority are not living in (and do not wish to be living in) full-time dominant-submissive relationships. Of those who are, only a tiny fraction have crossed the uncertain line into internal enslavement. This means that our experience is anything but typical, and we're out front about that right here.

Our experience of Master/slave is atypical in other ways as well. We are certainly different from the majority of people who do D/s, or M/s, or internal enslavement, in many ways. While we are not certain of the exact sexual preference statistics, most people are heterosexual, so we can probably assume that the majority group is straight here also, while we're pansexual queers in a same-sex relationship. Most of them are single-gendered; we're transgendered. For most of them, S/M (sadomasochism) is a good deal of the "glue" that holds their relationship together, and it may well have begun in the BDSM community as an outgrowth of kinky sex. While we've done our share of S/M, this is not true for us.

Most people in D/s relationships are in love, and that state of being in love is a foundation on which the D/s is built. Most of the rest are simply not in love. We are in love with each other, but our love has nothing to do with the M/s, and the M/s is independent of it. Most D/s and M/s couples (like most couples of any sort) are monogamous; we're polyamorous. Most D/s couples use a lot of "traditional slave protocol", and we don't. Most D/s couples have a lot of negotiated limits set by the submissive; we don't. Most live in urban or suburban areas; we live on a little homestead farm in a tiny rural town. Our reasons for doing this, too, are often in the minority.

So if we're so anomalous, why should anyone care about what we have to say? Well, for one thing, it's important to have diverse voices talking about these things. Far too often—at least on the subject of lifestyle enslavement—the main voice describing how these things should be done is … porn. Bad porn, too, more often than not, straight out of the fantasies of writers who have never lived this life. The next loudest voice seems to be all the people who are desperately trying to copy the porn. The small remainder consists of M/s practitioners who are all very different from each other in style and approach—and that's a positive phenomenon that we intend to add to. If nothing else, our anomalous voice is a practical, thoughtful, experienced counterpart to what's already out there. Take it as a complementary path, and take what you will from it, if you find anything useful.

Our other reason for bringing up all our "levels of difference" is to drive home the point yet again that lifestyle enslavement—and especially internal enslavement—is absolutely not the One True Way. We don't recommend it to everyone, or even most D/s people, any more than we could recommend that they all run their sexual practices and preferences, gender expressions, geographical choices, and everything else the way that we do. Don't try to be us. Be yourselves, whoever that is, to the best of your ability.

That said, this is a peek under the hood of our machine, to see how it runs. Maybe it will give you some ideas as to how to build, or fine-tune, your own.

Definitions

These are our definitions for the purpose of this book. We realize that they may not be other people's definitions, and that there are large divisions among D/s practitioners as to where the lines are drawn, which we will touch on. No matter what lines we chose, we were guaranteed to offend someone. That said, we had to come up with something, or it would have been too confusing. So these are the definitions that will be used throughout this book:

Power Dynamic: A relationship structure with deliberately inegalitarian power distribution. Some people use the term "power exchange", but others dislike the word "exchange", as they feel that the power goes one way rather than merely being exchanged. We prefer "power dynamic" and will be using that term in this book.

Top vs. Bottom: This is referring to S/M play, and anywhere you see it used in this book, that will be the case. The top is the active partner in S/M play, and the bottom is the one who things are done to. These terms can also be used as verb forms—e.g. "to top someone" or "to bottom to someone".

Dominant vs. Submissive: This is referring both to personality traits (as in "it's not very dominant to be passive-aggressive at your submissive" and to chosen roles. The dominant is the one who is in charge of the situation, be that an hour-long scene or a lifetime. Since these words also refer to personality traits (usually differentiated by such language as "being *a* submissive" as opposed to "being *the* sub in that scene" or something similar) we believe that one can be a dominant or a submissive while still alone and unpaired. In a D/s relationship, there can be as many limits set by the submissive as the dominant is willing to go along with. The level of D/s can range from cursory to limited and specific to deep and broad, but there is generally an understanding that the sub is bound only by their word and could walk out at any time, should they wish to do so. We will sometimes use the term "honor-bound voluntary submissive" to differentiate them from an IE-type slave/property.

"Domme" is a term for a female dominant, but not all female dominants use it, especially since it has a "femme" quality. More butch (or at least less femme) woman dominants sometimes prefer "Master" or "Sir". In complement, "Dom" refers specifically to a male dominant. When it comes to genders in general over the course of this book, we've tried to alternate them for both subs and dominants.

Master/Mistress vs. Slave: These are the most controversial terms, the ones that people argue over fairly intensely. "Slave", especially, is a term that is bitterly fought over in various areas of the BDSM demographic. We've heard definitions of the word "slave" that are as varied and contradictory as this selection:

❖ Slave and submissive mean basically the same thing.

❖ A slave is someone who wants to be a slave, and self-identifies as one, regardless of whether they are actually in a relationship with a master/mistress. You can be a slave for just a couple of hours in a scene.

❖ You can't be a slave unless you are in a relationship with a master or mistress, any more than you can be a wife or husband if you're unmarried.

❖ "Slave" refers to someone who considers themselves to be owned, or "property" (however that is defined), while "submissive" refers to someone who considers themselves to be "in service".

❖ A slave is doing it full-time, 24/7, while a submissive is part-time.

❖ "Slave" refers to someone who is primarily service-oriented; "submissive" refers to someone who is primarily control-oriented.

❖ "Submissive" refers to someone who is primarily service-oriented; "slave" refers to someone who is primarily control-oriented.

❖ Slavery has nothing to do with how often you do it, or what your service-orientation is. A slave is someone who has voluntarily given up most (or all) of their rights, while a submissive is someone who still retains most (or all) of their rights.

❖ A slave is someone who has been psychologically altered (with their consent) to the point where they are no longer able to disobey; if you can still disobey or leave, you're a submissive.

❖ A slave is a nonconsensually owned human being in a slavery-condoning culture or subculture, who would probably rather be elsewhere. All humans who have consensually offered themselves in this way are not slaves, and should be calling themselves submissives, and their insistence on the word "slave" is disrespectful to real slaves.

Similarly, we've garnered contradictory definitions for the word "master":

❖ "Master" is the title for a male dominant; "Mistress" is the title for a female dominant.

❖ "Master" is the gender-neutral title for a dominant, applicable to either sex; "Mistress" is a subcategory title used by some dominant women, while others find it too reminiscent of "adulterous lover".

❖ While "dominant" is an inherent personality trait, the title of "master" is earned by convincing someone to be your slave.

❖ You can be a master without a slave; you need only be the sort of person who wants to own a slave, and thinks that they would be a good master.

❖ Being a "master" is about "mastery"; it's the ability to be competent (and in some versions of this definition, to be good at getting people to do what you want).

❖ A dominant is someone who has a sub in service to them; a master is someone who owns (consensually) another human being as property.

❖ Anyone can say they are a master or mistress if they identify that way.

❖ The title of Master (or, one assumes, Mistress) must be earned by acclaim from people in your corner of the BDSM demographic who have decided that you deserve it.

And so on. To be completely honest with all the confused people who are reading this right now, there is no great consensus in the various branches of the widespread and scattered BDSM demographic. There isn't even a consensus among people who take on those labels, and often there isn't a consensus among people in a single M/s-oriented group (of which there are few). We've seen some bitter and furious fighting over who has the right, or should bestow the right, to carry these labels. Sometimes this fight has driven people out of groups, or split groups up.

We have no wish to add to this kind of disharmony, but we're also keenly aware that no matter what definitions we choose, we're going to upset a lot of people, many of whom we like and respect. At this time in the ongoing self-discovery of the M/s and D/s demographic, there's no neutral ground with respect to defining yourself ... and especially others. So what can we do? (And more to the point, what should the bewildered reader who wants to settle on a definition resort to?)

What we're going to do is what we'd like to see happen in the various BDSM communities. First, we're going to acknowledge that the people holding every one of these contradictory definitions are doing so out of deeply held beliefs which are as important to them as ours are to us, and we respect those beliefs. We do not require people to believe that ours is the right definition, and we will respect the chosen titles of others out of courtesy, regardless of our personal opinions of the foundations of those titles.

Second, we're going to state the definition that we will use *for the purposes of this book*, because we have to use something. We will acknowledge that it won't be everyone's definition, and we're going to say up front that this is OK. We will encourage people who don't agree with our definition to mentally translate the terms in their head to match their own definition, so long as they are clear where we draw our boundaries.

OK, here goes. Brace yourself. *For us personally*, Master/Mistress and slave are relationship-bounded job titles, much like husband or wife. One can't really take on one of those titles without a necessary partner, and the same can be said for this pairing. These titles are not given out by a community, but decided on by the people in the relationship. A slave is someone who has voluntarily given up most or all of their limits for their master to hold, while a submissive still has most or all of those limits.

In terms of "consensual nonconsent"—for example, whether a slave who signed up willingly still has personal agency and can leave or disobey—we decided to go with a grey area on these definitions for the context of the book for reasons of reaching more people. We've tried to be careful not to assume for this minority practice in our answers, and to be explicit when we were directly discussing it. If we were referring to something that would only apply to Internal Enslavement practitioners, we tried to make that explicit. (For our definition of Internal Enslavement or Total Power Exchange, see the section on Internal Enslavement. We'll discuss this even more controversial topic elsewhere in the book.) We also decided to sidestep the gender issue of "Master" and "Mistress"; titles should be taken with regard to role and not to anatomy. (As far as we're concerned, if a male slave-owner wanted to call himself "Mistress" just on principle, we'd cheerfully go along with it.)

All right ... now, on with more definitions.

Owner vs. Property: These terms are used similarly to the terms above, but with the strong connotation that one party owns—fully possesses—the other party, with all the responsibilities that go along with owning something. In some circles, the O/p tag has been adopted by those who feel that the M/s tags are quickly becoming meaningless due to the vast numbers of part-time fetishists calling themselves "Masters" and "slaves".

Scene: There are two meanings to this word, and no real way to get around either of them. The first meaning refers to a single discrete episode of BDSM play ("...I got beaten pretty hard in that scene we had last week..."). The second, usually differentiated by calling it *the* scene, refers to the greater BDSM community in one's given area ("...switches seem to abound in the scene around here..."). Unfortunately, members of a wide variety of other subcultures also refer to what they are involved in as "the scene".

Munch: Informal term in the BDSM community for practitioners getting together nonsexually for a group outing, usually to a restaurant.

Protocol: A set of rules about the behavior of a Master/slave couple (or more than a couple). Protocol can cover everything from how people are to speak to each other to how people are to move their bodies. "High protocol" generally refers to a relationship with extremely formal behavioral interactions, whereas "low protocol" has more casual interactions. Protocol does not necessarily refer to ethics, morality, or how the household is to be run on a daily basis—for instance, "You will greet me by kneeling and placing your head between my boots" would definitely be considered protocol, whereas "This is the kind of laundry softener that we use" might not.

Random Acronyms:
BDSM: Bondage/Discipline, Dominance/Submission, Sadism/Masochism.
M/s: Master/slave
D/s: Dominant/submissive
M-type: Master or Mistress
D-type: Dominant
s-type: slave or submissive
IE: Internal Enslavement
TPE: Total Power Exchange

All other jargon is defined in the question where it resides, because we felt that it was most effective there.

Motivation and Attitude:
Masters and Slaves

Getting Started

Q: How do I find a master, or a slave?

Raven: Honestly, I have no idea. I'm sorry. If you're religious, I suggest that you pray that one be sent to you. That worked for me.

Seriously, if I was on my own and really looking, I'd put the word out via my friends in the BDSM demographic, and ask them to matchmake for me. They would at least have some idea who I was and what I wanted, and would know better than to suggest someone totally unsuitable. I might also go to events, or be on email lists/forums, without the apparent intent to "hunt". While there, I'd do my best to come across as an extremely honorable, thoughtful, courteous, and articulate dominant (or conversely a polite, helpful, sensible, and self-aware submissive). Establishing yourself with a good reputation first helps.

Joshua: If you're not having any luck in the local scene, or there isn't much of one where you live, you might try personal ads. Some people have success with personal ads, but one generally has to sift through a lot of unsuitable responses. Women placing personal ads will almost always get responses from men who don't seem to have read anything in the ad itself, including such things as whether she is a domme or a sub, or whether she is a lesbian. Personal ads are usually better at getting one no-strings-attached sex partners, but sometimes good relationship hookups happen.

Keep in mind that people who aren't your preferred type but who have compatible ideas about your preferred lifestyle can make good friends who can refer you to someone right, as well as give you support.

Q: Isn't the best place to look for a serious D/s partner the BDSM scene? At least there you can find out via the grapevine whether someone is safe, right?

Joshua: You'd think that it would be the best place, and certainly many people have found their match there. However, there are many reasons why a potential master or slave might not get involved in the local leather scene in their area. Even if time, money and accessibility are not an issue, the local leather scene might or might not have a heck of a lot to offer someone looking for a slave.

I also question whether involvement in the public scene demonstrates that a person is serious. It only demonstrates that they are interested in real-time human physical interaction of some sort. That desired interaction might be getting a blowjob from a girl wearing cuffs and a collar; or putting on lingerie and getting a spanking; or watching strangers do pervy things so you can masturbate to it later (or right then); or showing off their gear, skills or partner; or getting face-to-face emotional support for one's online romances. If we were to rate "seriousness" on a one-to-ten scale, I might say that the public scene is composed of people who are above a four, while the online scene is composed of people above a two.

Are folks in your local leather scene serious about M/s? Should one even expect them to be? Most folks in the BDSM scene, in my experience, are fairly serious about liking kinky sex and fetish gear. The local leather scene is great for these people. They can learn techniques, meet like-minded perverts, and buy new gear. They have a space to play with new people in public, without many of the risks involved in going home with them.

If you are lucky, you might find a group in your area that is specifically geared towards M/s (MasT—Masters And slaves Together is the one national organization aimed at self-defined M/s people), or your local leather community might be more favorably disposed to M/s relationships than most. Some BDSM communities, however, are firmly against serious M/s. Certain segments of the leather community, for instance, made it quite clear to my master that "real" BDSM is about careful, consensual kinky sex and role playing between equals, and that holding real-world power over someone on an long term basis was inherently abusive or delusional. To them, it should never be more than a sexy fantasy. By their definition, a "slave" is a boyfriend or girlfriend who enjoys being treated in specific submissive ways when they are in the mood for it. While they have the right to hold their opinions and definitions (as we just discussed in the introduction), obviously this is not an environment where it is productive to look for a full-time slave or an owner.

Sometimes people who do serious D/s or other forms of edgeplay get a reputation for being "dangerous" in leather communities that are less supportive of such things. However, sometimes people also get bad reputations due to doing stupid and reckless things, so it's best not to make the assumption that anyone classified "dangerous" is necessarily who you want to be chasing after.

The online scene at least gives folks the potential to meet people beyond their immediate local area, people who may or may not be involved in the local scene. Online it is much easier to focus in on people who have your specific interests and ignore those who don't. But either way, it can be a long and difficult search and you just have to pray that the universe sends the right person your way.

Q: How should I behave when I come to a BDSM group as a new sub?

Joshua: Once you find some kind of organization, it always helps to volunteer. It gives you something productive to do, rather than sitting by yourself looking nervous. Even better, it lets people see that you are the sort of person who'd rather do something productive than sit around. That gets noticed by the right sort of dominants.

There may not be a lot you can do at a BDSM social meeting (often referred to as a "munch"), but it docsn't hurt to ask. At a workshop or party, see if they need help setting up chairs, arranging snacks, hauling equipment, or watching a door. Just don't make a pest of yourself if there is nothing they want your help with, don't turn your nose up at "boring" jobs, and don't go fishing for praise.

It may seem simplistic, but when entering a new scene it is best to be unfailingly polite to everyone you meet. Fawning over the most important-looking or most attractive people while blowing off everyone else isn't going to win you any friends. Even if they aren't folks who you have any interest in playing with, word gets around, and you may misjudge who the "influential people" in the scene actually are.

Q: I'm a 19-year-old guy—will people think I'm too young?

Joshua: Some will, but unless you are looking for folks who are specifically into young people, there is no reason to make a big deal about your age. You can learn a lot from older folks in the scene, but they often become uneasy if you keep reminding them that you are closer to their kids' ages than their own. Just act mature and responsible and don't make fun of the old folks' taste in music.

Women in your age range are in *very* high demand and short supply in most BDSM scenes, so if that's what you want, it may take a while. There are a few BDSM groups that cater to "youth" in some urban areas; they're usually called TNG (The Next Generation) groups. If you are interested in older men or women, say so directly, or they may assume you aren't. Some older female tops tend to go for younger men, and gay/bi male tops are often very interested in a young man. For a submissive, playing up the "boy" thing in a sexy way can help folks see you as "fresh meat" rather than "inexperienced kid".

Q: I keep putting my profile up there, and no one answers! I'm a desperate young man who needs some kinky sex now! What's wrong?

Joshua: I suspect a big part of the problem is that only a very small percentage of the BDSM scene is actually looking for no-strings-attached kinky sex with random attractive young men. In my area, most of the folks in the local BDSM scene who are looking for casual hookups are only looking for kinky SM play, not actual sex, or at least they are wary of getting involved with someone who seems to be just looking for sex. You might have better luck in venues for folks looking for casual sex in general, and let it be known that you are a pervy bastard who likes this, that and the other thing.

I notice, looking at your profile, also that you've listed yourself as both a top and a bottom, and checked off nearly every interest on the list. Personally, I can appreciate someone being very versatile and open-minded about activities, but to some folks if a person is eager for any sort of kinky sex whatsoever with men or women, top or bottom, etc. then they might look a little indiscriminate or indecisive. You might do well to make one or more *specific* profiles, showcasing a particular aspect of yourself. Pick something that really strikes your fancy right now and make a profile that is focused on that. If you are hot for boots, make a profile under a name like "UKbootboy20", with pics of you doing naughty things with boots, and yummy descriptions of boot worship. It is all about advertising. You want folks to see your ad and get hot.

Q: <<i WANTS MISTRES REEL BADS!!! i AM A WORM!!! FLOGG ME NOW!!!>>

Joshua: I think you might need to work on how you present yourself. In your profile you come across as whiny, desperate and self-absorbed. That is never good. The only real information you give is about the sexual fantasies you hope your "mistress" will fulfill. Women online are flooded with emails and messages from desperate men who want them to play out various elaborate sexual fantasies. If that is what you want, see a professional.

If you are looking for a position as a full-time slave, approach it like you would if you were applying for a job. There is plenty of advice out there about interview and resume skills. Look it up. It all applies here. This is just a different sort of job.

On the off chance that you're actually looking for a real slave position, you're going about it the wrong way. In this case, what you should be looking for is a part time non-sexual service position. Think of it as an internship. Finding a 24/7 live-in position right off the bat is really unlikely. Offer to come by for a few hours to do some kind of *useful and non-sexual* service, something that has *nothing* to do with kinky sex or your domination fantasies. Wash her dishes. Chat with her, tell her what you are looking for. Be charming, polite, and entirely focused on her wants and needs. Your sexual fantasies have absolutely nothing to do with this. If you are young, you'll need to impress her with how mature you are. Show her you are useful and sincere and a quick study. Show her why you'd make a great slave.

What skills do you have? What are you good at? If a mistress in your area is in the market for a slave boy, why should she pick you? Experience isn't the only thing a mistress might be looking for. What sets you apart from the teeming hordes of would-be male slaves? Can you cook? Can you clean? Can you fix computers or cars? Don't focus on the sexual side of things. No one who is serious about finding a slave is going to pick some random boy off the internet without some incentive!

If you really have no selling points, delete your profile and go work on that for a year or so. Make yourself into a valuable and desirable piece of human property. Take some classes at the community college or a vocational school. Have something to offer.

Q: What should I do on an interview with a domme?

Joshua: The advice I have heard from female dominants regarding potential male submissives seems to come down to this:

❖ It isn't all about you. Think about what she wants, not what you want her to do to you.

❖ Don't think with your genitals. Don't talk about anything that turns you on unless she asks about it, and even then, keep it brief and factual.

❖ Show respect. Not groveling or drooling, but respect. Be neatly dressed, on time, and attentive.

❖ Under no circumstances should you intentionally misbehave in the hopes of a kinky punishment. Not even a little.

❖ If she has kids, don't act like they are a nuisance. Make it clear that you will not behave in front of her children in any way that she does not feel is appropriate.

❖ Do not send her unsolicited photos of your genitals. If she asks for a photo, send a flattering fully-clothed photo.

Female dominants seem to have the most trouble finding a man who genuinely wants to submit to them and not to his own fantasies. So do not expect her to be dressed up in a way that arouses you, or for things to lead directly to sex or SM play. If she asks about your qualifications or skills, do not launch into a discussion of SM or sex play. Many female dominants appreciate a man who can cook, do housework, yardwork, basic auto repair and home maintenance, or grocery shopping. Some like an attractive well-dressed man who will pose as their charming and polite "boyfriend" in non-BDSM situations. Very few are impressed with a man who talks about how wonderfully he performs oral sex, or how he likes his balls tortured.

A certain percentage of female dominants want a submissive who believes in the inherent superiority of women, but some are offended by this, so it is good to know where they stand before you open your mouth. At the very least, you should be familiar with the social and political obstacles facing women in this society, and appreciate the difficulties of being a dominant woman outside of the dungeon. Any female dominant is likely to be especially displeased with a man who goes on about how women are superior so long as he has an erection, but couldn't actually care less about the issues women face day to day.

Q: What skills should I learn in order to attract a master or mistress?

Raven: Here are my top favorites, things that would make me sit up and take notice in an interview with a submissive:

❖ Massage.

❖ Cooking.

❖ Housekeeping.

❖ Car maintenance and (ideally) repair.

❖ Doing people's taxes.

❖ Fixing things around the house.

❖ Secretarial work—making appointments, keeping a calendar, home office work, etc.

❖ Some sort of part-time work that can be done from the home for money.

❖ The ability to become engrossed in whatever the dominant's hobbies are.

You'll notice that I didn't even go into anything sexual or fetishy here. I'll leave it up to you to decide why. However, I can guarantee you that if you had everything on that list, you'd be a heck of a lot more valuable.

Joshua: The most important skill to learn is to be adaptable. Practice changing who you are—it doesn't matter in what way so long as you break away from what you want and think of as "you". You can start with trivial things. Take up a hobby and learn to enjoy it. Now take up a different one. Now take up one that bores you, or makes you uncomfortable, or involves associating with people who you'd rather not associate with, or is something that you just can't imagine yourself, with your current identity, doing. Change the way you dress—not to something slutty and slavey, but just to something different, something that will change the way people perceive you. If you start to think that this new look is the "real" you, change it again, to something entirely different. Change from your usual preferences, arbitrarily. Roll dice instead of choosing for yourself. Don't be a martyr; genuinely try to enjoy it and find the good in it. If you don't like it, learn to deal with that. Understand what a small thing it is, and accept it with grace.

Do not try to change yourself into the perfect slave, or think you even know what that is. You can make educated guesses, but you can't ever know until you are there. When you shape yourself into exactly the sort of slave you want to be, it makes you less flexible, not more so. Give up your attachment to who you are and what you want.

Do this a few times and you learn that who you really are has nothing to do with those things that you've been changing. This is all about making yourself into a vessel that can be filled with whatever your future owner wishes. You need to actually do this to understand it. You can hear or read this and think you understand it, but if you haven't done it—really done it deeply and lived it—then I promise you, you don't understand it. It isn't something you can understand in your head. So go try it out—the best trait any slave can have is adaptability.

Q: Would schooling make me more valuable as a slave? What sort of education would an owner want me to have?

Raven: I just arranged for my slave to go through a truly grueling period of higher education towards a degree that I decided he should get. I came up with funding, encouraged him, and did without while he went through a demanding 72-hour-a-week program. I feel that it was worth it, because he now has a career he likes instead of one he merely tolerated, and sometimes disliked. It was a matter of helping him reach his potential ... because that potential was something that would benefit me.

Above and beyond the point that this will all depend on your choice of master (and the assumption that you *won't* choose one who wants to relegate you solely to a house-slave, not that there's anything wrong with that per se), there is this question: How will this degree benefit a future owner? Will he or she be able to take advantage of your higher income? Will there be job security, if you have a doctorate and perhaps a job with tenure or flexibility? Insurance your owner could share? A way to support yourself if it doesn't work out? Similarly, how will this future education and the career that it leads to inconvenience a future owner? Long hours? A need to be closeted? Inability to get obvious tattoos?

Make a list of the advantages and disadvantages that this schooling, and the career that will follow it, will create for the theoretical owner. Then look for an owner who values the former and doesn't mind the latter. You might also start thinking ahead to how you could cut down on the disadvantages before they come up. If this is a particularly demanding school program, maybe you'd want to wait to look for an owner until you're done with it? It's better to wait and be able to give them your full attention than to have to cheat them for some years, as it were.

Joshua: Whether it is education or anything else, I don't think it's a good idea to put your life on hold waiting for the perfect situation to come in to your life. Build yourself the life that is fulfilling to you and brings out the best in you. If you make partner-hunting your full time occupation, it's too easy to settle for someone inappropriate just for the sake of having found someone. It makes you desperate, and that attracts all the wrong people. Besides, a desirable piece of property is one that can find better things to do with their time than cruise munches and answer personal ads.

Regardless of where you work to start with, think about working from home; perhaps doing contract or client-based work. You can work flexible hours and it won't eat your life unless you let it. The corollary is that any job that expects to be your number-one priority is probably not the best direction for someone who wants to be in service, because service is going to be your number-one priority. So long as you keep that in mind, it shouldn't be too much of a problem.

Also, remember that a degree—even a general liberal-arts sort of degree—and the college experience that comes with it can broaden the mind and make you more interesting. Some (although not all) dominants prefer their submissives to have similar educational level to their own; if you're looking for an educated professional, a broadly cultured education can be a selling point. This is especially useful if you're a sub who is looking to be more "decorative" than useful; remember that high-class courtesans were always well educated. Study history, art, modern politics, etc. While some masters might prefer a poorly educated, "simple" slave, they usually aren't the sort of masters that I'd want to get involved with.

Keep in mind the way the decisions you make now would affect a potential M/s relationship, but don't be sitting there waiting for the right person to come along and hand you the life you always wanted. The only thing I'd hold off on is having children or getting married. Almost anything else you can put down.

Q: I'm 18, new at this, and I want to own a slave. I know I'm not ready yet, but where should I start learning skills that could help me learn to be a good dominant? There's no leather community in my area; are there any real-world skills that would help?

Raven: You know what I'd suggest as a good exercise?

Babysit.

Seriously. Especially sit for older kids, the kind who don't need their diapers changed, but may need you to break up fistfights—carefully. Understanding clearly (because you've negotiated with their parents) where the edges of your authority lies, what you're allowed to do and not do. (That's good practice too, because it gives you experience in negotiating authority with adults who have emotional vested interests.)

I'm not saying that adult subs are children, nor that they all need parenting. But there are a sizable number of skills in common that carry over. At least I found it to be so. Especially the basic concept of being *fully responsible for another human being every minute of every day, without a break.* That's a *mindset*, not a thing you just do when you think of it. Responsible for at least managing, and sometimes actually providing, that person's physical (right food, enough sleep, medical care), mental (stress, psychological issues), emotional (feeling safe and cared for) and spiritual (fulfillment as a person) needs. Are you up to that?

The second thing that you can do is to get yourself into a position of leadership. If you can't find a job that will put you there, volunteer at a non-profit. There are plenty of non-profits who will jump at someone who says that they want to take responsibility for certain tasks. Interest groups are also good for this. Leading a group of adults who are not emotionally involved with you will give you good practice in (again) negotiation, walking your talk, proving your trustworthiness, and making good decisions. Your judgment has got to be better than average if another person will be following it devotedly. Start on non-devoted people.

My third suggestion is that as soon as you can, find people who are doing this for real, and talk to them. Ask questions. Watch. Get mentoring. There are a lot of M/s folks who live quietly and don't go to leather events, because their focus isn't on sexual activities so much as on lifestyle decisions as a whole. They're out there. Look, discreetly.

The fourth item, and most important, is that you have got to get your shit in a pile yourself. Are you more emotionally stable than the average person? Are you reasonably financially stable? Have you worked through most of your issues? Are you independent of all poisonous ties to past trouble? Have you thought through, clearly and methodically, what it is that you want from a slave, and which of those desires it is reasonable for you to expect? Have you checked with real-life people to find out how realistic your expectations are? You can't control someone else psychologically unless you have thoroughly explored and are entirely in control of your own psyche first.

Start with all that, before you even begin looking for a submissive.

Q: What if a master or mistress wants me to move in with them, and I want to do it as well? How should I deal with my current life?

Raven: These are my suggestions:

1) Take your important papers and give them to a friend that you trust to hold onto for a minimum of a year. Get official copies of them for yourself. If things go terribly wrong in that first year, it means that you can get to them if you need them. Eventually, if things work out with your owner, you'll be turning them over, but it will be the mark of a sane and patient and rational dominant to be able to wait as long as it takes for that, while you both take the time necessary to figure out

whether your living together is going to work out. (This might include some money, in case you find yourself unemployed and needing to relocate.)

2) If your dominant can make it to your house, pull everything out where they can see it, in neat organized piles. Have them walk through and point to anything they care to point to, and say, "Get rid of that. Keep that." If there are sentimental objects that you aren't ready to give up, they go to the abovementioned friend in a well-labeled box. You may be allowed to have them later, or if this turns out to be permanent, you can have the friend dispose of them then. Have a yard sale or giveaway of everything that the dominant doesn't want.

3) If you're moving long distance and they can't come to your house, you can send them an itemized, well-organized list of any belongings that aren't personal to you (like clothing, toiletries, meds, etc.) and ask them to check off anything they would rather not have show up at their house. Or, if they're the patient type, you can bring it all, lay it out in the driveway, let them go through it, and then you take everything they don't want to the local thrift store. Some dominants have their newly relocated submissives get a box in a storage facility, paid up a year in advance, and put their stuff there in case things don't work out.

Joshua did a major giveaway before he moved up here, so that everything he brought fit in the back of my small S-10 pickup truck in one trip. That was my limit. Some of that stuff was then further sorted upon arrival (and his computer did not survive the trip). But you want to keep your belongings to a minimum.

Also, if you are taking any ongoing medications or receiving medical treatments, you should give your new master/mistress a list of them, and what conditions you need them for, what they cost, and what sort of doctors you will require for them. This is only reasonable if they are to take charge of your body, whatever that entails.

Joshua: Originally, my arrangement had been voluntary service, not slavery, and prior to entering into the relationship I disposed of most of my possessions as I saw fit. (Not because I was going into service, but because I don't like having a lot of stuff.) Mostly I just packed up the few things I wanted to keep, and let my friends know that they could take anything they wanted. I had already given my ex all the furniture and housewares when we split up, plus whatever else he wanted. A friend snatched up everything else with resale value and sold it on eBay. Some of the stuff my master might have liked to keep if I had consulted him, but there was nothing he would have wanted all that badly. He was just glad I came up with suitable clothing for farm work and a New England winter. The rest he didn't care about so long as it fit in the truck. The only furniture I brought was a nice leather rolling desk chair, which promptly broke, if I recall correctly. My computer—the only remaining possession of "value"—broke in transit. While I wasn't exactly happy with that, it was somehow symbolically appropriate.

Q: Should submissives put a value on themselves? Or is that hubris?

Raven: A smart submissive looking to be owned *should* have a self-value price; just not necessarily a monetary one. They should decide how that value means that they deserve to be treated, and stick to that. To say, "I have a price—I am worth X amount of kindness, consideration, honorable treatment, etc." is what a would-be slave *ought* to do. Submissives who will desperately sell themselves to the first dominant-looking individual who comes along, without any thought to their self-worth ... get what they deserve.

Some dominants would say that submissives are priceless. I would say that I am a cynical old bastard, but to me there are more slave prices on my list than "priceless". To me, the list is:

❖ Not worth the trouble

❖ Maybe worth it if they can be changed enough

❖ Worth the effort more often than not

❖ Totally worth every iota of time and energy that I put in

Dominants should be consumers too, and not shop while desperate.

Q: I want to be a slave, but my husband doesn't want to be a dom! How do I make him dominate me? I've been kneeling at his feet whenever possible, I've been calling him "Master," I've been saying, "This girl would like to serve her lord and master," but he just doesn't seem to respond in the right way.

Raven: Oddly enough, this is one of the most common M/s questions of all time. The predicament of someone who is in a committed monogamous relationship and realizes that they crave some aspect of D/s and M/s in their lives may be even more common than those who are single and searching for the right dominant or submissive. It puts them in a heartbreaking place sometimes, and the above question is representative of hundreds of other similar questions we've seen. The answers are never easy.

To the questioner: The first problem is that you're talking about an explicit and protocol-based power dynamic—meaning that you expect your husband to take up new ways of acting. You want him to act in explicit, obvious, perhaps even stereotypically dominant ways; things that hit your buttons and make you feel "slavey". At least that's what it sounds like.

To me, trying to _make_ someone "act domly" is neither very submissive nor very effective. If he acts like a dominant because you want him to, and he wants to please you because he loves you, who is serving who? Who's in charge here? Who's running the show? That's what it sounds like to me—you are trying to "mold and shape" your husband into being the perfect

Dom of your fantasies. This is hardly being of service to him, nor is it giving over control to him.

(I'm just imagining being some poor shmoe whose heretofore unsubmissive wife turns around one day and says, in essence, "Honey, I want to be your abject slave. So start acting like a master! Honey, you're not acting masterfully enough. Honey, c'mon, I want you to dominate me in just this way. Sweetie, why are you watching TV when you could be dominating me, your abject slave? Hey, put down that remote and start dominating me, damn it!" I'm sure that's not the dialogue that's actually going on in your house, but are you sure that it's not the internal dialogue?)

If what you want is to extend the sexiness out of the bedroom so as to get more of it, great. But you won't be able to do *that* 24/7. Sex does not make 24/7 go, and if you really want to be a slave, the first thing that you have to let go of is the idea that the relationship will be run the way you want it. It won't. It will be run the way he wants it, whatever that is. That's the *point*. And if the way he wants it is that you guys do BDSM in the bedroom, and on occasional weekends, but during the rest of the time your service to him consists of being the perfect wife and letting him have his way to watch TV or whatever—well, then really being of service to him would mean, that's what you do, even if it's totally unsexy. That's an *implicit* power dynamic, meaning that even when it's not obvious, you are basing your decisions and actions around what you know to be his desires, and not yours.

A real power dynamic does not have to be constantly explicit in order to be constantly implicit. In fact, it doesn't *ever* have to be explicit, actually. Which might mean that the best thing you can do if you really want to be a slave is to stop needling him and let him have things his way, observe his habits and do things to make his life easier (not just things that make you wet to do) and learn to entertain yourself and keep yourself on track so that he doesn't have to spend all his time paying attention to you and your need for attention. If this isn't possible or emotionally fulfilling for you, that's not your fault, but it does mean that you're going to have to make some hard decisions.

You can't force your husband into taking control of you. If he's not the sort of person who does that naturally, then it's you who have to give up control—and that means giving up trying to control what the D/s will be like. It may take him years to figure out how he wants the D/s to look. If you really want to be of service to him, help him figure this out in a way that doesn't push him to do what you want just because he loves you, and then go along with it even if it's not at all what you had in mind.

In fact, if he has a long-standing habit of doing things for you because he loves you, that may be hard to break. If he's going along with your desire for him to act all dominant out of love, sooner or later that will become resentment, especially as it becomes clear who is getting their needs met and who isn't ... and that it isn't the so-called dom who is setting the tone for the relationship. And, in the end, if he doesn't want to be your full-time dominant, you can't make him.

Being a slave means that it's not all about you—or your fantasy, or your comfort, or even getting all your needs met. If this doesn't appeal to you, if you want to retain the right to advocate for getting as many of your needs met as he gets, I suggest that you refrain from 24/7. Just be his part-time submissive, or play partner. It is also true that an egalitarian spouse might be someone that you'd happily choose for an egalitarian relationship, but might not be a good fit for a D/s situation. This is likely to come down to those hard decisions I mentioned, on both your parts—perhaps polyamory and "outsourcing" the D/s, perhaps a breakup, perhaps giving up on the idea of lifestyle D/s.

Joshua: Now that Raven's given the bad news, I'll find some positive things to say. I understand why this sits wrong with people who are strongly naturally inclined to dominance and the people who are or desire to be in service to them, but I think I understand what kind of situation you are talking about.

I have seen folks who very genuinely wanted to serve their partner in some way attempt unsuccessfully to interest their partner in "dominating" them. It often goes badly, because the partner goes through the motions and never really latches on to the idea of actually being in control. But unlike being a submissive, I think that a great many people can enjoy receiving service even if it isn't their natural inclination or training. Getting them to that point may be tricky—even if the spouse has some motivation to take control, they may not have the experience to control another person successfully, or the confidence that they can ask for what they want and get it. If the would-be submissive is new to all this, it is likely they are going to struggle with certain aspects of obedience and motivation. So they both need training wheels.

Generally a submissive who wants to serve has been randomly throwing potentially submissive behaviors at the potential dominant in the hopes of pleasing them, and their opposite number is trying to be pleased by them. We can assume that if they are seeking guidance, then this isn't working well for either of them. The submissive has to stop this and give the dominant space to decide what they really do want, while still encouraging change in the direction that *they both* have enthusiastically agreed they would like to try exploring. (Otherwise, things fall back into old patterns.) So they both encourage and remind each other of the direction they want things to move in, and they continually reinforce each other's behavior. If the submissive is the one who is the most motivated to change the relationship in this way, then they are going to be the one who is doing the most encouraging.

Eventually, they will find their level. With encouragement and support from the submissive, the dominant will take the level of control they are interested in taking. If the dominant is inclined to take full control of the bottom, then *when they are ready* there will come a point where all the smiling or pouting in the world won't push the dominant any further than they are willing to let themselves be pushed.

But if it doesn't start out being emotionally fulfilling and pleasing to both people, it isn't going to get anywhere. From personal experience, I think that if a couple like this tries to start out too "hardcore", what they are likely to wind up doing is encouraging the would-be dominant to vent their petty sadistic urges and resentments on the submissive, who has no preparation for being able to submit in a healthy way to that kind of treatment. It goes to a bad place for both of them.

A stubborn, willful submissive will not be enslaved by the method I've described here unless the dominant is a quick study and more suited to this role than they'd previously realized, but I think that under the right circumstances a more pliant person could be brought under control in this way. People are surprisingly prone to becoming what they act like they are and what you treat them as if they were.

Q: I'm trying to get my husband to be my dom, and he says that he wants to, but he just keeps doing things that make me mad! The other day I asked him to go to the store and get some skim plus milk, and I had to nag him for ten minutes, and then he got the wrong kind! When I have to nag him to do things and then he does them wrong, I feel like I'm the dominant and he's the submissive!

Joshua: No, if he were the submissive one you could simply tell him what sort of milk you like and he would get exactly what you asked for. The fact that you had to pester him for several minutes before he could appreciate that you see an important distinction between "skim" and "skim plus" milk shows that he is most definitely not submissive to you. Really, no reasonable person has ever suffered terribly from having the "wrong" sort of milk to lighten their coffee in the morning, so he likely underestimated what a fuss you'd make over it.

Masters often do small things to indulge their slaves' various whims, but they do them as they choose and in the manner they choose. They may have a certain motivation to please the slave, but not being submissive themselves, they don't place the same emotional importance on doing things exactly as they are told.

However, many masters will also do things to shut their slaves up when the slaves are making pests of themselves. That might arguably not be in the long-term interests of maintaining discipline, but many masters seem to settle on what level of obedience they require and don't exert themselves to enforce a higher standard than that. If they aren't the sort of person who takes a special satisfaction in training and disciplining a person, there is a point of diminishing returns in this sort of thing. After that point, the master could make the slave more perfectly obedient, if they chose, but on some level they've decided that it isn't worth the hassle.

To the slave, how obedient they are is one of the single most important things in their world, so it can be hard to accept that their master might not want to perfect their obedience to the highest imaginable point. The master honestly may not notice or care that the slave took thirty seconds longer than needed to come when called. (If they do, they are almost certainly the sort who takes a great deal of satisfaction in training.) An extra thirty minutes is a problem, but thirty seconds? Some masters (mine, for one) don't care if there is some minor foot-dragging or private eye-rolling involved so long as what needs to get done gets done.

And there comes a certain point where a person, slave or not, has to accept that how they feel is under their own control. The most effective response to the thought, "When Master does X, it makes me feel un-slavey," is to think, "How can I keep from feeling un-slavey when Master does that?" Getting the master's help on the matter doesn't meaning persuading them to not do X—obviously, figuring out how to make your master do what you say is counterproductive in trying to achieve an appropriately submissive mindset.

What the master might be able to do is discuss their motivations and reasons behind their actions to help the slave see how their actions fit in to the power dynamic. That might be as simple as the master saying, "I'm not going to censor my every word or action for your benefit. It is your job to do things in the way I find appropriate, not the other way around."

Q: I want my wife to be my slave. She likes to bottom, but doesn't want to go further. How do I convince her to become my slave full-time? I've started by rewarding slavey behavior on her part and ignoring her when she's not submissive enough. Will this work?

Raven: You've answered your own question, unfortunately. Your wife gets into the idea of temporarily pretending to give up control, because she still really has control—she asked for it, and she can stop it whenever she wants. She doesn't want it to be real or full-time. For her, it may be a sexual fetish, not a lifestyle.

While that may be inconvenient to your goals, there's actually nothing wrong with that. Most people are on the side of it being a sex thing, not something that they want all the time. Just because she gets turned on by a fantasy during sex does not mean that she wants to give up power over the breakfast table ... and, frankly, it's wrong of you to try to push where she doesn't want to go. If you keep that up, you will probably lose her, unless she is so codependent that she will eventually go along with it unhappily anyway and just be miserable, and that's not what you want.

I understand because at one point my wife was sexually hot for bondage and play-submission and all that as well, and we foolishly tried to make it a full-time thing. It didn't work, and it created a huge problem that took months to work through. We both felt betrayed, in different ways. I had to accept the fact that for her, it was a fun sex game (and now that her libido has declined, she's not even really interested in that any more) and for me, it was more than a game. We resolved it by my agreeing to keep our relationship entirely egalitarian, and I got myself a secondary lover who is a natural slave. In other words, I outsourced the D/s. Obviously, if you two are sworn to monogamy and polyamory is out of the question, you've got a problem. But you might be surprised ... if your wife realizes that this is important to you, and that she really doesn't want to give it, she may be glad to have someone else relieve her of it. But you'll have to very careful ... first, not to make her feel bad that she is not cut out to give this to you, and second, if you get a slave, not to fall so madly in love with the dynamic that you forget to pay the proper attention to your wife. Those are the two dangers I've stumbled over as well.

It's hard, I know, to know that you have this deep need inside you to take part in a D/s relationship, and your partner doesn't ... but that's life. Outsourcing might be a possibility in these situations. Either that, or divorce, but I would not throw away a loving marriage over this one need unless there was no other choice. In the meantime, by "rewarding" her for submissive behavior, what you're actually telling her subtly is that her normal and preferred way of being is not good enough. You're also playing a head-game on her without her knowledge or permission. That's not a good thing.

The Owner: Ego and Responsibility

Q: Why did you want to own a slave anyway?

Raven: I should first disclaimer that I am not claiming that my reasons are typical, or even likely to be that of anyone else. They are simply my own. They also aren't very flattering, but being as I'm the guy who goes around talking about owning your own monsters, well, so. I expect it's up to me to be an example and lay it on the line here, too. In my twenties, I felt that being a sadist was terrible and wrong, and I tried to purge that from myself, to no avail. Eventually I discovered the ethical solution of doing this with consenting people who would ask (even beg, sometimes!) for it. The same goes for this situation. If you can't get rid of the urges, is there an opposite number out there for whom it is a Good Thing?

There are several reasons that having a slave is emotionally important and fulfilling to me. First, I am an extremely possessive and territorial person. When I love fully, all the way to the wall, I want to own someone completely. Since I also juggle polyamory and egalitarian relationships, this means that I am always holding back that last little bit of myself with them, because they don't want to be the focus of the predator who wants to piss on them and declare them to be territory, to be hoarded and defended. (And I don't blame them. It takes a special person to want that.) So having one person in my life who wants that, and with whom I can be that "monster", makes it possible for me to be generous and egalitarian with the others in my life.

Second, as I will discuss in the Internal Enslavement section, there is great comfort in that kind of commitment, and it's that territoriality gives me the ability to commit. Well, actually, it's not so much committing as locking on with iron jaws and never letting go no matter how much they scream and wiggle. Letting go of that which I love is not easy for me. M/s allows me to be as obsessively committed as I want to be, as it is in my nature to be. It gives me great comfort to know that he is that committed as well—because there was a point where he consented to this, after a long time and a lot of discussion, with full knowledge that he would then be permanently bound. It's an equally obsessive commitment, if you want to bring equality into it. Someone attempting to tell him that he ought to leave me will find that this soft pretty boy has a sharp, biting tongue and knows how to use it. Not to mention that the transparency involved makes relationship discussions *much* easier! No lying, no holding back, no hiding one's agenda, no careful dancing around the point, no having to put things a certain way so as not to damage someone's delicate feelings and have them flounce off! Just cut to the chase and get the work done.

Third, and even more difficult: I find it very, very hard to be totally emotionally open and vulnerable to someone. I used to deal with that by just not doing it, or only doing it partway. I don't trust easily, and I am a control freak. Obviously—I have non-M/s relationships—I can open up 75% of the way when I love them, although it is excruciating in many ways. But in order to be completely open with someone, they have to be rendered entirely harmless as far as my subconscious is concerned. That last 25% just won't happen unless my lover is first made totally vulnerable to me.

I realize that this reason, above all others, will make some people cringe and feel that there is something really wrong with me. Maybe there is, but I've been working hard on myself for many years, and this (like my urge to territoriality and being an alpha) just does not seem to go away. So the options are to either not do it at all or to find a place to put that, too, which M/s gives me. I also realize that some dominant-types will not understand why I would possibly *want* to open fully and vulnerably to another human; after all, it isn't very stereotypically "domly". To them I say: poo. I can use my slave for anything I want, even as a place to be safely vulnerable. If the slave has a problem with that, they're not a suitable slave for me.

Fourth, well, I just enjoy the selfishness. I enjoy that I have a relationship where the other person is willing to become whatever I want as a partner, within their ability to do so without damaging them mentally. I want a relationship where it all goes my way, or at least where all the important parts all go my way. I am a very selfish person, although I am also intelligent enough to not let that out where people who won't appreciate it (which means everyone I don't own) have to be burdened with it.

Most people, of course, want a relationship where all the main things go the way that they want it. Instead, they must compromise with another human being who wants the same thing, and there will be power struggles and arguments and all the other things that are part and parcel of learning to have relationships. As someone who is also is an egalitarian marriage, I agree that those things have value. However, in having a second relationship with an owned slave, I give myself a place where I can be far, far more selfish than any other relationship would (rightly) put up with. It gives me a place to put those urges, and breathing space to recoup and go back to the (more difficult) egalitarian relationships refreshed and ready to give what must be given. In return, the responsibility of my slave's well-being is a tiny price to pay for a luxury that most people never get.

It's the same logic that I use about polyamory. I am emotionally incapable of monogamy, so my options are cheating, celibacy, or ethical and negotiated polyamory. The first is unacceptable to me for ethical reasons, the second for emotional and physical ones. All the time and effort and negotiation that goes into successful polyamory is entirely worth it in order to reap the rewards of getting your needs met in an ethically clean way. Far more, than worth it, actually; a small price to pay. Ditto M/s.

And fifth, it's just more practical. My life is complex and difficult, dealing with three jobs and a chronic illness, and I need to know that I have someone who will do what I say, especially in emergencies, without argument or delay. It is comforting to me on a practical level that I have an extra pair of hands who are very much an extension of me, given the delay in communication that being required to speak rather than just think does create. I'm able to do much more and be more effective in the world with this human extension of my will.

Q: Have you always known that you were a Master? When did you figure it out?

Raven: I've always been an alpha, from the very beginning—willful, showy, intense, and controlling. That didn't mean that I always acted like one—or was allowed to. But inside myself, I was going to be the one in charge. Whenever I was in a situation where I felt that it was possible, I took control of the group and ran things the way I thought that they should be run. Like Peppermint Pattie and Marcie, I secretly wanted someone to follow me around and call me Sir, and carry my stuff, and fetch for me, and occasionally let me hurt them. My first sexual fantasies were power-based as well.

In the fourth grade, a boy named Jim was poking around the girls on the recess ground pretending to be a cow. He'd "Moo" and try to poke his nose up under their skirts. So I suddenly decided (to this day I can't remember *what* was going through my head, it just happened) that I would tie him to a tree with a jump-rope to stop his bad behavior. He laughed the entire time and didn't try very hard to stop me. Then once he was tied up it suddenly occurred to me (what *was* I thinking!) to whip him with my jacket. This only made him laugh more, and a crowd was attracted by his "Mooo! Ha ha ha...Ow! Mooo..."

Then the zipper on the jacket got him in the eye and blackened it—what can I say, I was eight years old, I hadn't had safe S/M training!—and we both got sent to the principal's office. I was terrified I'd be suspended. Jim laughed the whole time and told the story to the principal complete with mooing, and the man shook his head and kicked us out with a warning.

(Someday I am going to run into Jim in a leather club, on someone's leash. Then I can wave and say, "You don't remember me, but I was your first dom...")

On the other hand, from a very young age I was subjected to a great deal of abuse from two mentally ill parents. They both put a huge amount of work into attempting to break my will and make me compliant and pliable. Some of that work was emotional, and some quite physical. I endured regular beatings and worse for small (and sometimes imaginary) wrongdoings on about a weekly basis until I finally ran away at the age of 17.

Did they break me? No. They did screw me up pretty good for some years afterwards, though. It took quite a while to work all that out, and during that time I stuck to vanilla egalitarian relationships, because I didn't trust myself. As I grew up and healed and came into my own power, I wanted more and more to be not just the one in charge, but the one in control. At the time, I felt this was terribly wrong of me. After all, I'd seen firsthand what happens when people who *want* to control you are allowed to, right? It took yet more time to convince myself that power didn't necessarily automatically corrupt, and that it didn't have to corrupt me. Starting BDSM—which was control for small periods of time—was a way to get past that, to show myself that no matter what they had done to me, they had not completely poisoned me. I wasn't like them. I could be in control of someone else and not harm them; I would never lose it over someone's vulnerable body. My self-control, in those situations, is flawless ... because it has to be.

After years of doing BDSM, where the scene ends and everybody's egalitarian again, I found M/s—and had to start all over again with deprogramming myself, convincing myself that wanting this—wanting it with a hunger that ran deep and hot and hard—wasn't just a symptom of being a selfish and inconsiderate person; wasn't just something that I would be spiritually better off purging from myself. As I said before, it's what you do with an "unacceptable" urge. Find a place, however narrow, where it can live, and try to learn to love it anyway. If you can't love it, well, maybe someone else can ... someone who loves that in you. And, if possible, harness it into the work of redemption.

I had "done time", as it were, in the feminist, nonviolence, peace-activism, ecological communities. I still work with those folks, and try to build bridges, but some things about myself I no longer discuss with them. That worldview strongly implied that no human being ought to have the kind of mastery over another one that we here are talking about. Not just because no one could be safely trusted with it (according to that view) nor just because it would be "bad" for anyone it was done to, but also because it was just something that people oughtn't to have, because it would screw you up and make you sociopathic, or at the least irredeemably selfish.

So in spite of all this ... a childhood where two people constantly attempted to beat me into being submissive, and then years of political discouragement ... I found myself unable to uproot these urges. Sure, I could live without a slave; I could live with that hole in my life. There are a lot of holes in our lives. We deal with them. So, OK. Put it aside and let it be.

Except that then I prayed and asked (in separate prayers) the Powers That Be for A) another lover who was the same gender as me, B) assistance in my work, C) emotional support, D) someone to take care of my health needs, and E) commitment. The Gods saw fit to deliver all of the above in the form of a beautiful boy with a malleable personality ... and then, before we knew what we were getting into, we realized that he was getting enslaved, and we talked about it and agreed that it was a good thing.

So if it wasn't what I'm supposed to be doing, why was it quite literally the answer to my prayers?

I realize that it is also a test, and a practice. It's not just Joshua that I have control over. I'm a leader of other groups of people, and in influential positions with still others. I'm a writer, and have the chance to shape minds. Enslavement is a particularly intense and hands-on version of "ordinary" leadership, where mistakes count triple and you'd better not screw up. This is spiritual training for responsible leadership in the outside world. I do occasionally wonder if my horrid childhood was somehow arranged so I would never forget what it is like to be on the low end of a power dynamic with unworthy people in charge of your hapless ass, and always retain that compassion.

Now, it feels comfortable. Natural. Dependable. It's still difficult to justify to people who don't get it, but it's where I am. I will always be an alpha. What I do with that is my own choice, and that of people who choose to submit to me or not.

Q: What are different kinds of owners like?

Raven: There are a variety of ways to categorize owners, all of them very subjective and prone to argument. For example, I once compared owners of humans to owners of cars. I suggested three separate categories, although I know that there are probably more than three. This is what I could think of offhand as a good metaphor.

There are work-oriented owners who want a slave to do specific things to make their life more comfortable—someone service-oriented, practical, proactive, self-sufficient, motivated, who can take both directions and initiative. The car equivalent of that would be the person with the rugged four-wheel-drive all-terrain truck that can drive up mountains, gets awesome gas mileage, is incredibly reliable and has a really good warrantee, and probably a trailer hitch, a PTO, and a bunch of useful racks to hold tools and extra lumber. The sort of thing that could tow someone else's stuck vehicle out of the mud without so much as grinding the gears. If it gets a little dinged up, you fill in the scratches with nail polish and go on.

There are owners who make a hobby out of managing their slave—perhaps the word "hobby" isn't intense enough, perhaps part-time or full-time preoccupation (or avocation) would be better—owners who want extreme obedience and malleability, someone who can adapt well to being moved around like a puppet in all areas of life and like it, often to the point of almost total dependency and maybe never leaving the house. The car equivalent of that is the guy with the classic car that he works on during weekends (and on every other minute that he can steal from the rest of his work), refurbishing it, messing with it, upgrading it, constantly improving it. Likely he only takes it out of the garage for special drives and to show it off. The point isn't an immediate goal of perfection (or even real-world usefulness) but the joy of the process of control and creation—how far can I go with this project?

There are owners who want a beautiful and sensuous pet who will curl up at their feet and look adoringly at them, who needs to be protected and maybe reassured a lot, maybe even a trauma sufferer who needs healing, but who is so fetchingly and vulnerably submissive. This is like the car owner with the expensive upscale sports car with the leather interior and the gorgeous custom finish—maybe it needs to go in to the dealer frequently for maintenance and expensive repairs, but there's nothing like the feeling of privilege and sheer luxury when one reclines in the perfect climate-controlled padded heaven and sails gleefully past the slower barges. There are probably other sorts of owners too, who could be compared to other sorts of cars, but these seem to be the most obvious of the lot.

Another way of classifying dominant styles is to place them on a continuum from what could be called "parental" to what could be called "celebrity". The "parental" style doesn't have to have anything to do with ageplay; it's just a style where the dominant is heavily focused on taking close control in daily activities. The "celebrity" style is more about the dominant receiving service, and helping the sub to render them more perfect service. Most dominants will fall somewhere in the middle, but it's instructive to look at the far ends in order to get an idea of the situations. As an example of both, picture a nice restaurant where two M/s couples are entering, sitting at separate tables, and ordering dinner.

At the far end of the "parental" style, the dominant drives to the restaurant, orders for the submissive (because they know what's best for them), pays for the meal (because there's no reason to let them touch money), makes them eat everything on their plate, decides when to leave, and then drives them home. It puts the submissive in a childlike role in a lot of ways—protected, supervised, getting things done for them, control maintained by not allowing them access to "ordinary" independent adult things.

In the "celebrity" model, the dominant is chauffered to the restaurant by the submissive, who then goes in and picks the best table while the dominant makes calls on their cell phone, and orders the food for both of them (because the submissive knows exactly what the dominant wants to eat, and what the submissive is allowed to eat), and the dominant might not walk in until after the meal is ready and on the table. They eat until they are done and then get up, regardless of whether the submissive is finished, and the dominant walks out leaving the submissive to pay and tip, which they don't want to be bothered with. In this model, the submissive is more of a devoted servant/assistant whose job is to make the dominant's life free of all annoying details.

I've seen both types among all gender combinations, although some seem to be a little more common than others for certain genders. It may also be a matter of who the dominant uses as an example of power: the people who first had power over them as a child, or the people who had power over those people?

I am very much at the celebrity end of the spectrum, although it took me a while to realize that this was what I really wanted. Because of being the eldest child of chronically ill parents, I had a great deal of pseudo-parental responsibility as a child, and when I became a dominant as an adult, I assumed that the parental style was the way to go. (I was also an actual parent at the time, which contributed to this idea.) After years of being that sort of dominant, and attracting the sort of submissives who want that sort of dominant, and being generally unhappy with the situation (although not so unhappy that I was willing to give up all but egalitarian relationships), I realized what I really wanted to do and started looking for the appropriate servant. Which is a lesson that beginning dominants should take to heart: Until you're sure how you want it to go on your own terms, you won't attract the right people for those terms.

Q: What does it mean to be "worthy of service"? Isn't that a subjective thing?

Raven: I agree that the answer is subjective ... but it's still important, even so. It's very important to me that I find myself worthy of another human being giving their entire life over to me. In my mind, this is a privilege. I grew up poor, and I'm still not well off, and so having a slave is an amazing luxury that I never expected to have. Yet here is this person whose whole life has been derailed in order to cater to me. In order to be worthy of this privilege—not worthy of *him*, but of the privilege of owning him, or anyone for that matter—three things must happen.

❖ I must not fail in my code of behavior, in my honor with regard to my dealings with my slave. This means treating him and his service as well and fairly and rightly as I can.

❖ I must help him to perfect his own path of service, and value his path as well as my own. This means helping him to find his way through what I ask of him, whenever I can.

❖ I must use him as best I can to perfect my own path, which means using the time and energy that he frees up to do worthy work in the world—and "worthy" in this case means that it makes a difference outside my own home. Every free moment that is created by his presence in my life must never go to waste.

I don't expect that all owners will hold themselves to this—heck, I don't expect that any besides myself will. But that's my subjective definition of Worthy for myself, applied only to myself. I've always seen having a slave as a privilege granted to me (by the Powers That Be, not by the slave) that I have to continually work to be worthy of. It's an ongoing price. If I become dishonorable, abusive, uncaring, or otherwise reprehensible, then I am no longer worthy of the privilege of having someone give up their whole life to follow me around and do for me ... and I would assume that the Powers That Be would relieve me of that privilege.

It's not just that I constantly work to take good care of my slave. It's that I am supposed to constantly work to be the sort of person who is worthy of dedicated service ... and that sort of person would, of course, take good care of their most valuable possession, but that's not all that they would do. To me, part of earning that worthiness is being worthy outside of this relationship as well. It doesn't count if I'm good to my slave but rotten to the waitress, the bank teller, my employees, my kids, people on the Internet, and everyone else who has less power and recourse.

Q: I'm tired of living up to my slave's expectations of me. I'm a pretty good person, and I try hard, and I'm sure that I'm not a bad owner, but my slave keeps expecting me to be perfect, and is upset—and frightened, and angry—when I'm not. This is damned unfair.

Raven: Oh boy, is this an issue.

It's interesting to put this question right after the last one, which goes on about how owners should strive to be better people, and here we are talking about how good they are "required" to be. I would guess that all the long-time experienced slaves I know could easily give you a list of their owners' faults and bad qualities. After all, they spend so much time studying them! It isn't that the experienced slaves think that their owners are perfect. It's that they don't need to be perfect. They serve them anyway.

I am an imperfect human. I like to think that I'm above average when it comes to ethics, morals, commitment, all that character stuff—if I wasn't, I wouldn't be fit to own a slave—but I am no cardboard cutout, and sometimes I screw up. I always strive, but sometimes I fall short. When I fall short, I pick myself up and try again. For some very hard things, or things that are currently very hard due to circumstances, I may fail repeatedly. That's no excuse for failing to continue to try, but in the short run it does cause problems.

This has been an issue with Joshua, because he's the sort that fastens on negativity and obsesses about it. (I've been working on changing that in him, but it's a long haul and we've not made much progress.) One negative experience has the weight, for him, of twenty or more positive ones. If something goes right fifty times and goes wrong once, he will remember it as not working and usually going wrong. I have seen years of good experiences with something literally wiped out by one bad experience with that thing where something went wrong, and it took years further to build up enough positive experiences to counteract that one negative.

This means that every time I screw up—which, as I'm human, is inevitable—it can be an emotional disaster for him. I'm not just talking about things that are directly related to him, or to enslavement; I'm talking about him seeing me screw up in any area of my life. The internal enslavement has progressed to the point where it isn't undone by this; it just makes him frightened because he loses trust, and angry at me for frightening him so when he wants to feel safe with me. His tolerance for any imperfection in my behavior is extremely low.

So the question is how much I, as an owner, should care about—and alter my behavior due to—my slave's opinions of me. Keeping in mind that trust can be damaged by the slave having a poor opinion of the owner, how much weight should the owner give to the slave's opinion of their behavior? Obviously, too much weight given and who's in charge here anyway; not the owner, that's for sure. But how much is too little? Where is that line? What about when the "who's in charge here" line is perilously close to, or even on the wrong side of, the trust line? It's a difficult balance to dance with. There's also that time is slowly helping him to be more comfortable with my imperfections, as he can see that things aren't all going to fall apart because that bill got paid late or I've been putting off trimming the goats' hooves for over a month.

Slaves are going to have expectations of their owners, because they need to know that they will be dealt with fairly and be made safe. No one (sane) wants to have their life and existence in the hands of an erratic nutball, or an incompetent idiot, or an uncaring sociopath. I'm not arguing that the submissive shouldn't have expectations that the dominant will be a decent person. Usually the expectation will be that the dominant will be *better than just decent*, because, let's face it, subs want to believe that their dominants are all better than average people—and in some cases, amazing, awesome people. But where is that line fair to draw? When are expectations too high, and a product of the slave's damage? How does one lower them without causing problems, or should one? How does one help the slave to deal with their feelings on being enslaved to an imperfect human being? And, most importantly, how much of the slave's expectations of how exceptional they ought to be will the dominant adopt and strive for in order to maintain the slave's trust? These are all questions that must be fought through in the dominant's mind—often in the wee hours of the night—and each will find their own answers.

The areas that are important that the dominant be "better than average" in will vary with the sub in question, and their needs, fears, values, and insecurities. One sub may need the dominant to make a lot of money and uphold a certain lifestyle, and will panic if they have a period of time where they are only making a subsistence living. Another may expect the dominant to be an utter paragon of perfect morality and go into a panic if they steal pens from the office. Yet another may expect the dominant to be constantly superb at manipulating, second-guessing, and outwitting them, and panic if they have a tired, depressed, unperceptive period where they handle the slave clumsily. Yet another may require that the dominant always be assertive, decisive, and "masterful", and panic when they decide to take a week and sit in front of the TV while tasks pile up.

I think that the need to see one's owner as a superior form of human (otherwise they wouldn't be worth submitting to, right?) can be very tempting to allow to escalate into expectations that would be considered unfair if they were placed on anyone else. That's where the pressure sets in, and that's where the dominant has to take terrible risks, deciding where that line needs to be drawn, and risking losing the slave's respect, trust, or actual presence either way.

But hey, no one ever said that this would be an easy job.

Q: Do you own a slave because you want to control your surroundings, or because you don't want others to control you? Is it about being the one who isn't controlled, but who controls others—or is it about making your environment what you want?

Raven: From what I've seen of most dominants, I'd say that we are all people who don't like to be controlled ... and I'd say that the vast majority take on slaves because it's one place where they can be in control of someone else who can't control them. But for myself, it's about controlling my surroundings. I've done a pretty good job of creating the surroundings I want—I can't carpet the world, but I've put down a lot of throw rugs. Of course, I don't like being controlled much either, but that's a losing battle for a lot of reasons. My religious practices require a great deal of discipline and very limited choices.

Having a slave is not a way for me to feel masterful, or highlight how I am the one controlling and not the one controlled. If I want that, I'll go speak in public and make an entire roomful of people feel a certain way. That's real power. Having a slave helps me to control my surroundings. The food I want appears before me. The sex I want happens when I ask. When I'm sick, help appears. The work I need done that I can't do myself, or don't have the time for, gets taken care of. Money appears in my checking account. My website changes magically whenever I order it. Pleasant companionship is always there for me. The affection I offer is never rebuffed. The affection that I get is offered in exactly the right way. I can start and stop any of it whenever I want.

Q: Should a master apologize to their slave when they make a mistake? Isn't that "undomly"? I feel uncomfortable when my master apologizes to me, and I tell him not to do it. After all, you wouldn't apologize to your other property—your sofa or mailbox, would you?

Raven: I say Please and Thank You to my slave just like I say Please and Thank You to everyone else. I feel that thanking people when they do something for you, and apologizing when you screw up, is an important courtesy in the rest of the world.

My slave is only one of the many, many people that I have to deal with on a day-to-day basis. Although I could let my habits of politeness slip with him, there is the ever-present possibility that this discourtesy would leak out and splash onto others who I don't own, and who didn't consent to be treated in that way … and that would be entirely unacceptable. So my verbal habits of courtesy are a kind of behavioral discipline that I set for myself, and breaking that discipline for my slave, just because I could do so without censure, is not good for me.

But then I've always been uncomfortable with the model of mastery that encourages masters to use their slaves as a way to coddle their egos and encourage thoughtlessly indulging reprehensible behaviors, just because they can.

Of course, there's a difference between using the slave as a place where one can behave reprehensibly, and using the slave as a space where one can let one's hair down. I make reference to the latter in many of these answers. The difference is that in the first example the master/mistress has decided to dispense with acting honorably and responsibly, and in the second they've merely decided to dispense with the sort of considerate niceties that require one to censor one's self for the sake of the feelings of others. The first is more poisonous to the master/mistress than most of them would like to admit. The second is simply a way of venting. It's up to the intelligence of the dominant in question to make sure that the latter does not slide into being the former.

Joshua: When my master has screwed up, he's very up front about it. I'm not at all required to pretend he's always right. He routinely thanks me and says he's sorry, if only because he does not want to appear to be treating me rudely in front of random witnesses. Even if we're alone he'll do it out of habit. I wouldn't say he ever asks for my forgiveness, though. He just expresses his regret over what happened or acknowledges his error. Aside from being a genuine expression of gratitude, my master thanking me is part habit, part maintaining an appropriate public image, and part acknowledging whatever I did. At its most formal, his "thank you" means "That will do," or "I am aware of that."

Actually, his "I'm sorry" can also mean "I am aware of that", especially if he's just done something that inconveniences me. It can also mean "I didn't intend to hurt you in that way," "I know it sucks; do it anyway," or "Your complaint has been registered. Drop it."

Sometimes when he's sick he'll ask me to do work he normally does, and he sometimes apologizes for that at length. That used to make me very uncomfortable, but I'm getting better about it. In part I think he does it to express his regret that he cannot do it himself. It isn't really about inconveniencing me or asking my forgiveness. He has to keep his emotions in very tight check in much of his life, including in his personal relationships, and part of my job is giving him a safe space to express however he's feeling and be uncensored. If he had to act a certain way around me to keep me from becoming offended, he wouldn't choose to spend nearly so much time with me. On the other hand, he refuses to be a jerk, even in that safe space, and I can only respect that.

As for being uncomfortable with your master apologizing, since when is it a slave's place to decide what are appropriate things for the master to say to the slave? You have to look at what is going on in the head of a slave who is so uncomfortable with their master saying they are sorry. It is one thing to hold the opinion that your master needn't apologize to you for anything he or she does, and quite another to beg to not ever be apologized to or claim it is inappropriate for the master to do so.

Really, even if a master doesn't think they owe the slave any apology, who is to fault them for giving one? If you can say to your slave, "On your knees, you filthy cunt-whore!" why couldn't you say, "Gee, I'm sorry I upset you yesterday. I didn't intend to." The master can say whatever they damn well please to their slave.

True, most people don't apologize to inanimate objects, but slaves aren't inanimate. Besides, if you did apologize to your mailbox, your mailbox wouldn't get pouty about it.

Q: We've been doing this master/slave thing full-time for a few weeks now. My slave has been serving me, and I've been enjoying it. But this week the shit hit the fan—she got sick, we had visitors, my job kept me late—and I told her to stop serving me and treating me like her master until she's better, the people are gone, and I'm through this week's work crisis. I feel like a failure, like I couldn't keep it up and had to go back to an egalitarian thing. Am I being too nice? Am I a weak dominant?

Raven: When I was first messing about with this dominance thing, I think that one of the hardest things was not knowing what my "style" was supposed to be, and thinking that I had to be something besides myself in order to do this right. That was incorrect, and a product of too much BDSM porn, and too many other dominants trying to tell me how I should be doing things. I eventually learned that my "style" could be whatever I felt like at the time, so long as I was the one setting the tone, making the decisions, authorizing the action, and committing to lending my best judgment to the situation.

Being dominant doesn't mean that you can't be low-key, or gentle, it just means that you Get The Job Done. Above all else, though (and this is something that new dominants are prone to doing, especially if they love their subs and want them to be happy) your decision as to which mode you are utilizing at any time *cannot rest on what your sub would like you to be doing*. It has to be what *you* think is the most effective style for right now, even if they don't like it.

With egalitarian partners, before D/s, I often found myself subtly manipulating things so as to go my way, and of course I couldn't say that I was dominating the situation. When I first embarked on D/s it took me a while to admit that A) I'd done that a lot, B) that was part of me wanting to be in charge, and C)...why, here I didn't have to do that, I could just say, "Actually, this *is* how I want it to go, and this is what you're going to do, because I'm In Charge Here." Once I got it, once I understood that I could just Say It, and it was Real ... oh, my, the freedom in not having to constantly step on that urge.

I don't know you, but I suspect it's possible that the Too Nice danger zone is probably about you not owning your own managing of the relationship. Deciding unilaterally that We Are Going To Stop With D/s Play For A While Until I Say Otherwise isn't egalitarian, my friend. It's being in charge. And this process of owning when one is controlling the tone of the relationship, whatever that is for the moment ... is the process making talking D/s from something that you "play" or "do", and making it something that the two of you *are*, all the time, implicitly when it's not explicit, even when you both look like you're acting absolutely normal. It means you're starting to make it Real.

Oh yeah, one last tip: As this process happens, expect resistance from the sub. That's normal too. The resistance may even come in the form of them telling you that you're not being dominating enough. That's them crying, "This isn't the fantasy that I expected! This is ... too real life!" That may end in deciding that real life isn't what is wanted, or it may end some other way.

Q: I've got a demanding job, and I want to find a slave who can cope with periods of being alone while I'm working. Will this just make the slave feel taken for granted?

Raven: From a purely practical view of this topic ... I've found, in practice and in my observations of others, that when a slave complains that they are being taken for granted, what they are really saying is: "You aren't paying enough attention to me."

I think that's really the root of the fear: if a slave is too good at their job, if they just become the machine that creates the perfect life for their owner, will the owner get busy paying attention to that life, and not to the slave? The answer is variable ... some masters might, some might not. Some slaves are content with a certain minimal level of attention, and others need more.

It's one of the questions that I advise potential dominants to ask potential subs: what is the minimum amount of attention that you need from me, per day or per week, before you start to feel like you're not getting enough to be anything close to emotionally satisfied (not to mention properly enslaved)? I also warn them that unless they are dealing with an experienced sub who's been through more than one live-in full-time situation, they will probably not get an accurate answer. It's one of those things that s-types don't know until they go beyond that line. If they've only had vanilla or mild D/s relationships in the past, they're used to demanding attention—we all do, in non M/s relationships—and it may not occur to them what it will feel like to be told to do some virtuous occupation and get out of the owner's hair ... for an hour, a day, a week.

Generally, they will err on the side of saying, "I don't need that much attention." Because being needy is not good selling material, and everyone knows that ... and owners are all different as well. Some may put inordinate amounts of attention into their property, and want a certain level of neediness and desperation. Others may want more of the luxury of being able to ignore them for long periods and still have them ready and waiting when called.

So that's the big question that obliquely answers the issue of taking for granted ... how much attention do you need? There's also the attendant question of "how much deliberate validation do you need?" Those are a good calibration for what that s-type would consider being taken for granted.

I admit that I am biased in favor of a slave who is proactive and has good problem-solving skills. In my mind, that's what a well-trained slave *is*—one that you don't have to supervise all the time. Just like a well-trained employee is one who knows their job and does it without constant supervision. Right? Does an employee "self-boss", at least to a certain extent? Well, yes. The good ones do, anyway. The ones who don't are generally considered lousy employees.

Or ... perhaps the word would be "high-maintenance". And there are masters who love, and specialize in, taking on such subs. But obviously that wouldn't be right for you, so you will need to be up front about how much attention they will or won't get on a daily basis, and make it clear that you are looking for someone who is fine with that limited amount.

Q: Is it necessary to keep parts of yourself back from your slave, so as to create a veil of mystique? It seems that slaves really want to idolize their masters, and it doesn't seem like you can do that when you show off your grubby bits.

Raven: Well, it is easier to maintain control when you have at least some kind of emotional barrier up, and when you have a substantial portion of inequality in information—they tell you all their fears and worries, you keep most of your shit from them. It's not just about looking good, it's about not making dents in their confidence if they see you losing your shit. According to the people I've polled, many submissives (but not all) would prefer this. It helps them to keep trust in their owner having everything under control, not just them but *everything*.

Having said that, I then have to admit that I can't do it, at least not with a slave who is also a live-in partner and lover, and whom I have fallen in love with. One of the services that I want from my slave is to use him for emotional support when I need it. That's become far more important than I ever could have imagined. I have a lot of trust issues myself, and having someone to talk to about my shit who will always listen and engage with me, that's been a wonderful boon.

I've seen a lot of dominants do the whole "I don't need anyone to talk about my goddamn fucking *feelings* with, goddamnit!" Well, maybe you do and maybe you don't; whatever. But then I see an awful lot of them go skid-mark-sideways because they're so busy maintaining their facade that they don't allow themselves an outlet. It sneaks up on them and then they do stupid things. OK, so if you're busy keeping your slave impressed with you, find someone else to let it out on. A friend, a shrink, someone. Me, I'd rather use my slave, because I trust him more than anyone else in the world.

There's also the fact that this person is observing you in depth, constantly, desperately, in order to please you. (Or they *should* be.) And they're going to see a lot more than you want, whether you want them to or not, unless they are A) not really very bright or observant, or B) invested so heavily in that perfect view of you that they are deliberately ignoring what they see. I think most dominants who are doing the facade thing would like to believe that their submissives are a lot more fooled than they really are. I dislike the hiding game anyway, as it can lead to dishonesty or lying by omission. It's also a pain in the ass to have to remember to keep things from someone who's in your personal business all the time.

Joshua is a suspicious, slightly paranoid little Scorpio. He likes to know what's going on with me, because his own fears of what *could* be going on with me are usually far worse than anything that actually is in reality. So sharing with him paradoxically makes him feel more secure, not less. He has held me through many a meltdown (usually when I'm sick and in pain; battling chronic illness means that there will sometimes be days when the disease is dominant). The important thing is that he's also seen me keep it away from the rest of my life so that it doesn't splatter and affect external issues—and then get back up on my feet, get back in the saddle, and get on with things. He knows, also, that it will never get "bad" beyond a certain point—there is a certain level of self-control that will always be there.

That's how I've built his trust—not convincing him that I never lose it, but that when I do lose it, it will be discreet, contained, and I will recover from it, and it will not damage anything. In other words, that I'm still in control, even about my temporary loss of control. This also makes him complicit in helping me to get back up there in the saddle without other people seeing it, and makes us a team, not adversaries in the process. He knows what to expect, he knows what to do, and he knows that it works. That's what's needed. But this takes sanity and balance and good self-control in general.

Q: I've got a new slave, but I'm used to living alone and doing for myself. And I like doing the cooking and cleaning, but it makes her feel insecure that she can't do all those things for me. Is it unmasterly of me to want to do the laundry? After all, I know how I like it done.

Raven: Here's something you can do. Go through the chores in your head that you are used to doing, especially the multi-step ones. What are the steps that are least enjoyable and most grunt-work? Assign them to her. That way, you're still in charge of the operation, and you get the more fulfilling stuff, and she is there to help you.

For example—even if she's a good cook, you decide that you're making dinner tonight. Great. She can shred lettuce, chop veggies, wash pots and pans as you use them. You're the chef, she's the assistant. That's the key—think of her not as someone to replace you at these jobs, but as an assistant. You want to do the laundry? She can run down and put the softener in half an hour from now. You want to vacuum? She can move things around at your direction and put them back. She can fetch things for you, and hand things to you. It's actually good for her, because she gets to see how *you* want them done, not how she would prefer to do them, which is the big trap many subs fall into when they first move in. "Oh, this would be so much better if it was done this way, even though my dominant does it that way..." No. She should learn to do it *your* way. Letting her assist, and perhaps giving her a bigger part of that over time as you feel like it, will help with that.

Q: What about when the dominant humiliates the sub because it turns the dominant on? What if they enjoy seeing the sub as their inferior?

Raven: One person's humiliation is another person's good time, and hardly touches a third person's ego. It's a highly subjective thing. We're assuming, in this situation, that the humiliating things aren't being done to teach the submissive something—"...oh, you think that this job is beneath you, do you? Well, guess what!"—but is being done solely for the dominant's entertainment. We will touch on the issue of sadistic entertainment in the Punishment section, but for now I'll just say that the danger zone comes when the dominant's assumption that the slave is their inferior makes them mistreat the slave. That sort of person often mistreats those who fall beneath them in status, and I'd suggest steering clear of them as owners. However, if they treat their slave well but simply honestly consider them inferior to themselves in some way, that's different. A submissive who wants their dominant to enact specific behaviors to prove that the dominant sees them as an equal in some dimension had better pick a dominant who is fine with that. A sub who hates being deliberately humiliated ... ditto. It's a matter of fit.

Joshua: "Inferior" is a tricky word. I'm certainly my master's social inferior, and as I've said elsewhere in this book, I have a very difficult time serving someone who I don't see as better than me in some meaningful way. But I know that I am successful at what I do and that I am a good person. It isn't an issue of self-esteem, just an issue of status.

I've done humiliation play with a number of tops. With tops I liked and respected, I mostly felt like I was humoring them. Sometimes it was sexy, sometimes it was silly or uncomfortable, but not really humiliating. It is just service. It might embarrass me a little at first, but I find I can get used to damn near anything if I know it's serving and pleasing the dominant.

However, the few times I've done humiliation play with tops I didn't respect, I had a good deal of difficulty hiding my contempt for them. I can generally be very eager to please with a top who I don't respect much, but it is difficult if they want something like that. If it is humiliating, it is because it makes the top look like an ass, and I hate to be seen as someone who'd happily obey an ass.

I do get a certain sexual kick out of stereotypical slavey behavior, the groveling and bootlicking and whatnot. That is just a fetish thing, I think. It doesn't feel humiliating when I'm doing it; it is normal and it feels appropriate. It is my place to do these things, and I'm content with that place. In some ways it is very comforting to be used in that way. If I found that sort of thing humiliating, I think I'd be in the wrong line of work.

Q: How do you make decisions as a dominant about things that are difficult or painful for your slave? (Orders that aren't harmful, just something the slave hates.) How do you help them get through it? I'm worried that a dominant will simply try to force me through commands I don't want, and I'll rebel in spite of myself.

Raven: All right. I could use my boy Joshua as an example, but since your difficulties with the idea seem like very personal fears, I'm going to use a theoretical you. Let's say that you're my slave. (I know that's not easy to imagine because you don't know me that well, but let's just suspend disbelief here.) Let's say that I notice that you've been getting behind on the chores I've ordered you to do, because you're on the Internet all the time, mostly on blogs and lists and forums. First, I sit you down and we have a conversation. I tell you what I've been seeing. You tell me that your Internet lists are an absolute necessity for you emotionally, and beg me not to take them away. Do I believe you? Well, considering that I've been studying you for the past several months or years, I'll know when you're lying to yourself. I'll know that voice and that body language. (If you're someone who would consciously lie to me, then you'd have been weeded out in the first week, and the point would be moot.) So I'll watch that. I'll listen to your reasons for needing large amounts of time on the Internet. I'll judge them as to how specious they sound, and what I know of how your mind works.

I'm also probably wondering about whether I should give you an ultimatum—I'll let you prove to me that you can do all your chores without my cutting back your Internet time—or just say forget it, you get one hour a day and that's all. Which I pick will have a lot to do with what I know about you. Do you have time management difficulties that have required more supervision in the past? If so, I'm not bothering with an ultimatum. I know where that will get us—right back here again. If I do let you prove it to me, the first failure will boot you back to one hour a day, period.

For, you see, I'm not some distant general giving commands from on high, not knowing or caring whether they cause you pain. I'm the exact opposite. I'm in your head already. I know you like a book. I know every emotion that crosses your face. I've interrogated you about everything, watching, judging, figuring you out. You are not allowed to hold anything back from me, and I long ago learned how to wrest out those thoughts that you weren't giving me. I can second-guess you almost every time. I am waiting around every mental corner for you, always one jump ahead. And really, you don't want to beat me at this, because it is deeply comforting to you that I am always one jump ahead.

This is not distance. It's an intimacy so deep that most people would find it frightening.

So let's say that I know you have time management difficulties, and you've failed me before, more than once, when asked to schedule your day effectively. Let's say that I decide that the Internet is a cookie, not protein. Or, more likely, that it's fast becoming an addiction. that pulls you away from the important things. Free people have the privilege of fucking up their lives with addictive behaviors. You don't. You will be forced into healthiness whether you like it or not. I say so. Internet is down to one hour a day, period. And, in fact, I want you to take a week off, starting now. You can write one email or post telling people that you'll be away for a week. You probably feel terrible, and right now you hate me.

What do I want you to be thinking at this point? We will have discussed that. I'll have given you steps to take yourself through mentally in order to cope with a difficult order. The first one is to remind yourself that you signed up for this, that you knew that there would be hard things in among the good things. You will remind yourself, quickly, of what some of the good things are. You will remind yourself of why you signed up for this in the beginning, why it was the right choice for you.

Second, you'll remember my track record. You'll remember all the times when I was right and you were wrong, regarding judgments about life issues. You'll remember that I am better at this than you, and that's why you chose me. You tell yourself that it's very likely this is for the best, and that it's worth it to wait and follow my word and see if I'm right yet again. You step on the inner voice that wants to prove me wrong. After all, my being consistently wrong would feed your ego, but ruin your trust in me as your owner, and it would be all over. If I'm right, you're inconvenienced, but you're safe, because it's reinforcement that I'm worth obeying. That's a better outcome, so it's worth waiting for,

Third, when you've calmed down some, you think about my priorities, and consider this from my angle. After all, you've been observing me too, for months or years. You know me pretty well, and that's why you trust me. You remember how hard I work myself, how upset I get when I can't do my task because you've spaced doing one of yours that interlocked with it. You remember how pleased I am when we run smoothly, like a well-greased team, and everything falls into place. You remember what I look like when I'm pleased with you and with the life we've made together, and you desperately want to see that look on my face again. I know that this point will take a little while for you to come to, and that's all right.

In the meantime, I'm painfully aware that you're angry, and hurt. Don't think it doesn't run through my brain to say *never mind, go ahead, it's not such a big deal.* Except that it would be. If I did that, then every time that I was thwarted because of your Internet habit from now on would make me feel terribly resentful towards you, and it's not good for an owner to feel resentment towards their slave. That can lead to all kinds of badness. I'd also resent myself for giving in, and I'd feel like I wasn't really in charge ... and then we'd end up right back here. Better to do this now. Anyway, I can always change my mind later if it's really proven to me that you need it, or can handle it.

I give you a little time to yourself. Perhaps I give you an order to do something that you actually like, but that is useful to me. Not intimacy, not sex—you're angry, and I want to let you cool down. I'll pick a chore that you find fun, or at least that you're good at, that will reinforce the link between doing what I want and feeling good. Later I check in on you, ask how you're feeling towards me. If you've been having trouble getting through the acceptance process above, I help you with that. We walk through it verbally. I'm supportive of you and give you positive reassurance for getting through it.

The week goes by. I check in with you to see how you're feeling a few days into it. I want to know if you're obsessing over the blogs and posts you're missing; I'm looking for addictive behavior. If I see some, perhaps I start thinking about ways to get you more social contact that work within my schedule and needs. Perhaps I give you more attention. If this is a product of isolation, I want to do something about it. If it's something else—if, for example, I know you're prone to addictive behavior—I discuss that with you, and help you to see what I see. We talk about how you can deal with the Internet in a healthier way.

The week is up, and now you're back on the Net for an hour a day. I watch to make sure your chores keep getting done. I wait a week and check in with you again, see how my decision is affecting you. Is this enough? Are you adjusting to it? Is there anything that can be done to help you with that?

Of course, right now you're probably wondering: Under what circumstances would I rescind that order and agree that you really do need four hours of Internet a day? Well, let's say that the problem is isolation. Let's say, further, that I've accepted a job on a tiny station in Greenland and dragged you, my slave, along with me. You don't speak the language, you have no one to talk to but me, and I'm busy most of the day. At that point, I'd have to look at my own choices. I brought you here, and I'm responsible for your mental health. I can't tell you to not need contact, any more than I can order you to flap your wings and fly. My choices are to let you have lots of Internet and put up with fewer chores, to enforce my rule and have you miserable and close to a meltdown, or to move home. I can't have everything, and as a mature human being I need to accept that.

You may not always be aware of what's a need and what's a want, because your wants may feel very much like needs to you. It's my job to figure that out, from observation and experiment and deduction and intuition, and then I enforce it. I'll likely have made errors, especially in the beginning, but I will have made few enough that you trust me and my judgment to be better than yours. I know you better than you know yourself. Simultaneously, I'm constantly working to understand myself fully as well, so that no unconscious resentments or pettinesses well up and sabotage my handling of both our lives. You see that, and you admire it. It's part of why you trust me with this decision-making process, and why you can let go and let me tell you what to do.

Q: You've both mentioned in your workshops that the slave's biggest area of striving should be their attitude. (*Authors' Note: This is covered in the next chapter.*) **Is there an equivalent for the master/mistress?**

Raven: Yes. The counterpart of attitude is motivation. If the slave's job is to struggle to have a clean attitude, the master's job is to continually strive to command with clean motivations. A mindful and thoughtful M-type will be constantly working on their understanding of why they do and want and create what it is that they do, and making sure that their leadership does not come from a place that is petty, vindictive, malicious, insecure, or otherwise unworthy of them. They don't have to explain their every motive to the slave, but they had best be conscious and clear about those motives with themselves.

Q: My submissive said that she wanted X, and so did I—so I did it, and she freaked out and rebelled! What's going on here, and what should I do?

Raven: That's one of the most common problems new dominants have, I'm afraid. I certainly found that to be a source of screwups in the beginning of our relationship. It's inevitable, because the process is so delicate and we have so little guidance on it. It took me a long time to figure out that often—not always, but often—the internal unspoken dialogue around resistance is actually going like this:

S: I want to try this new activity of submission!

D: Great! I'd love that! Let's do it. (Goes ahead with plan.)

S: Ow! I don't like this! It's way more work and way less fulfilling than I thought it would be. I don't want to have to do it. Actually the thought of having to do it day after day makes my blood run cold. And it reminds me of how little power I have here. That's scary. Justifiably scary! My survival instincts are kicking in! But wait, I want to please my M and do this, I want to be a good slave, I want to achieve this new level! But I just can't seem to do it on my own, I don't have the strength, I can't make myself! The survival instincts are winning! What do I do? Aaaargh!! (This last cry comes out as a rebellion or meltdown.)

D: But ... you said that you wanted to do it! Oh, never mind then. (Is bewildered and feels betrayed. Either lets up, at which point S says:)

S: ...Hey, I feel let down. That's not what I really wanted. I wanted you to help push me through it. I think. Didn't I?

(Or D makes them do it anyway, in which case S says:)

S: I can't don't make me I can't don't make me I can't ... hey look, I can! I just needed help pushing past it.

The problem, of course, is knowing when it is the above situation, and when it is an actual serious problem with a command that is really bad for the sub in some way. That's so hard to tell in the beginning, and the truth is that in the throes of "Aaaargh!" the S may not be able to see that clearly. If they could, they'd probably have a better chance of doing it themselves. So the D has to guess, and hope, and use their best judgment, and pray that they're right.

And sometimes we err. I tended to err in the direction of giving up too soon and letting Joshua down, not having the nerve to push, and/or wanting very much to believe that he was always introspective enough to figure out whether it was a real crisis or just a bout of intense anxiety, and be able to tell me clearly every time. Taking his word for it every time meant that I often gave up when I should have pushed. And, once in a while, I erred in the other direction too.

The aftermath of those errors were a whole lot of talking to each other, deep processing, figuring out what went wrong on both sides. Over time, I slowly became more skilled at judging the situation, and could see the places where my own baggage had interfered ... and where his had. This processing has to be done together, not a "You horrid person, how could you!" on either side, but "This M/s thing is a team effort, so let's figure out together what we can do about it."

It helped Joshua to come to a point of humility, too. I think that humility in a slave is far less well summed up by "I am a lowly object, Master!" and much better summed up by, "Sir, I've thought about it, and I have to admit that I may not always know what I want, or what's best for me, or whether something is a need or a want, or whether something will damage me or not, and I won't always be able to give you clear information on that, and I'm sorry, sir, so I'm trusting you to figure it out." Assuming that there is that level of trust; if there isn't yet, neither one will get past the barrier. Work on building trust and giving the dominant a chance to learn the inside of a submissive's head better, and then go back to those boundaries and see if they're really so impossible now.

Joshua: Partly it depends on the activity. What's going on might be, "That looked fun from a distance until I tried it," but in some cases it could be "That's fun but only if I'm forced to do it." These tend to apply to kinky activities.

On the other hand, if it's a matter of self-improvement or deepening their slavery, that can be different. There have always been things that I want to be able to do, or believe myself capable of doing, if only I got the right guidance from my master. Usually these are personal goals that I've been trying unsuccessfully to achieve for many years. When a sub says "I want to do X" in this context, on some level what they mean is "I want to be able to do X", and they want to rely on their dominant's strength to help them achieve that goal. They know that their dominant has helped them to achieve difficult things in the past, and has more willpower than they do, and they are hoping that the dominant will apply this talent to the submissive's goals. If they were able to do it without assistance, they'd already have done it.

It can help if the dominant pries into the submissive's history of X and related activities, before the command or at the first sign of rebellion. Did they have problems with that sort of thing in the past? Where did they fall down in the process on their own? Are they just wanting to know how intensely the dominant wants them to do X? Knowing that their dominant is seriously set on a particular behavior can be a stronger motivation to them than they might have been able to summon up before this. (This, of course, hinges on whether the dominant actually cares much about the order, and has any interest in following through on it.)

Q: Do you do random "acts of dominance" on a regular basis to keep your slave feeling slave-like? Do you feel obligated to do them?

Raven: I'm rather a hardass on that. I expect a lot of self-motivation from my boy, I expect him to have a good attitude no matter how non-dominant I'm acting at the moment, and to remember at all times who and what he is. He does marvelously at this, and I consider myself lucky.

When we were first starting out and getting the hang of this—while I'd had several boys before him, they were all submissives and not psychologically enslaved—he would bring up needing more acts of dominance, and I'd try to do that in order to make him happy—it's maintenance, right? Got to do nice things to keep the slave happy, because happy property works better, right?

Nope. If I was doing those things primarily for his maintenance, they held no joy for me. And certainly no erotic power. In fact, I began to feel resentment about having to do things which I'd have been glad to do if it had only been my idea and only on my whim. And then I'd pull myself up and say, "What the hell? Who's in charge here? Screw this!" And I'd stop, and he'd be unhappy.

It's something that I have to keep in mind: selfishness makes me happy, and fuels my feeling of ownership. I am capable of being terribly unselfish—heck, I have to be in the rest of my life—but it is un-erotic and very emotionally unsatisfying. The more selfish I am allowed to be (allowed by my own ethics, that is) in any given situation, the happier it makes me. I spent decades trying to be different, to be more altruistic. Didn't work. I can act the part, all the way to the wall, but it only makes me resentful. My random acts of dominance have to be entirely spontaneous on my part, or it won't work for me. That's one of the things that I *need* a slave for—a place where I can be entirely selfish and it's still ethically correct—because my daily life requires a huge amount of altruism.

So what I had to do was to train him to respond to whichever acts that I happened to feel like doing at the moment, rather than the acts that he might want that day. Since he's malleable, this has worked well. We're working towards it being enough, on days when I haven't done anything to him at all due to being busy, that he remembers how he is supposed to behave, and that this behavior is not his choice nor what he would have wanted, and that will reinforce his submission.

This is something that I think comes later in enslavement, and it's when the real depth of it sets in for the sub—when whatever acts of dominance that you wanted have less of an enslaving effect than *anything* that your owner desires that you don't want. Knowing "This isn't the way I wanted things to go—and they're going the way my owner wants them, even though I hate that—and that means that I'm the slave, and that's paradoxically terribly satisfying to me!" can be a real eye-opener for a slave.

But I still do random acts of dominance; they're just done as generosity, not maintenance. One thing that I like to do, and that he gets practically every day, is to be idly fondled in various (often nonsexual) ways without regard to his personal boundaries, dignity, or whatever he's doing at the moment. I'll toy with some part of him in passing, and he's required to stay still and put up with it even if he's cooking on the woodstove and I've decided to fondle his nose or ears. I sort of treat him like a puppy or a doll in that way, and he's come to respond very strongly to that depersonalization and casual violation of physical boundaries. The fact that it isn't even sexual drives it home further. And it's something that I do every day effortlessly, so it's again less about me going out of my way and more about him adapting to what it is easy and comfortable for me to do.

But that was the gist of it—in order for that to work, he had to adapt to whatever things were convenient for me to do. Of course, he started out with the right attitude—a submissive who hated getting what they wanted if the dominant was only doing it to humor them or make them happy. From the beginning, he couldn't stand that. I think some subs haven't even gotten that far yet.

Q: What do you think about films like *The Secretary*, where the dominant forces the woman to do all sorts of things to prove her love for him? Is it romantic, or not?

Raven: I have probably read entirely too much ancient and medieval literature (meant in the sense of stories, not non-fiction), but whenever I see tales like *The Secretary* or other ones where the male dom puts the female sub through all sorts of trials that are not only difficult but downright dangerous, and doesn't seem to have much of a care for their well-being, yet the sub is supposed to go ahead and prove their loyalty again, whether or not the dom deserves it...

...I can't help but think of the tale of "Patient Griselda" in the Canterbury Tales, where the wife is horribly abused by her husband for years and all the while takes it passively and obediently, never complaining about her treatment. It was supposed to be a patently ham-handed "morality tale" about how good medieval Christian wives were supposed to behave. All the *Secretary*—type films and books look like a replay of "Patient Griselda" to me, sorry.

So, temporarily putting aside all the issues of safety or sexism or whatever, the thing that really bothers me is, as always, that the *dominants* in these stories are piss-poor role models. In "Patient Griselda", six hundred years ago, no one ever asked the question of whether it was good for the husband—morally or psychologically—to brutally abuse someone and have little regard for their well-being for many years, just because he could. Similarly, when people criticize the boss in *The Secretary*, they all focus on his dominance as the problem, not that he's a lousy and unsafe dom. In fact, I'd say that 99% of BDSM porn has lousy, unsafe doms as role models. Many are clearly insane. Others are simply neurotic in various ways that make their actions seem bizarre and senseless. (This is especially true of femme-domme porn; it's hard to find any where the domme isn't an irrational nutcase of some sort, which is an insult to female dominants everywhere.)

I understand that many people eroticize danger, and submitting to a sociopathic loony can be a hot fantasy for some people. I remember being told about one pro-domme who lost a lot of clients when she got sober, because they preferred to be beaten wildly in a drunken rage. But really, what are we teaching future masters? Not that we need to censor porn. But are worthy dominants so boring and pedantic that there's nothing worth writing erotically about them? What's going on that almost all portrayals of D/s in fictional media have awful dominants? For that matter, are the characters in fictional pieces like *The Secretary* actually morality tales, warning us that people who do this are dangerous?

The constant portrayal of D-types as opportunists with no self-control, no personal discipline, no greater goals, no regard for their slaves' well-being, no ethics, and no honor really disturbs me. Yes, I know this will be blown off as self-righteous whining by some, but I'm one of the dominants who actually attempts to help struggling "new" dominants. I see what the overwhelming majority of bad examples does to them— including creating a raison d'etre for people who actually are opportunists with all the above lacks.

Maybe I've just gone too far with this—it has gotten to the point where every piece of D/s fiction makes me ask myself, "What does this say to the world about the nature of D/s and how it should be done?"—but it pisses me off.

Q: Do you think of your slave as livestock? Is that a good comparison for live property?

Raven: I may be one of the few slave-owners who actually owns real livestock. So my view on the matter is necessarily different.

It's not that I don't give a damn for my goats and sheep (and chickens, ducks, rabbits, and geese) and it's not that I don't take care of them (I was just up all night a couple of nights ago helping a sheep birth out twins), it's that there is one huge difference between my livestock and my slave. If I decide that I don't want my livestock any more, and there's no immediate market for them, I will simply slaughter them and put them in the freezer and eat them. If they're not fit for human food, they'll become food for my dog.

Here, since we butcher out our own meat, killing and disassembling animals is a big part of caring for livestock. It takes up a lot of time. Even with breeding stock that I had grown attached to, when they got old or developed problems that would cost more to fix than I had (which isn't much), it was time for the bullet; if they are too sick to be eaten, they get cremated. Above all, They Are Food. Meat. I have the legal right to kill them, and I believe that I have the moral right to kill them quickly and cleanly after having given them a good life. (And no, I'm not interested in hearing whether anyone else thinks that I have the moral right to kill and eat animals. It's not germane to this book, will take up too much space, and that discussion doesn't belong here. Suffice it to say that I believe that I have that right, and that belief shapes my experience of human property vs. livestock.)

I do not believe that I have the moral right to kill my slave if I feel like it. (I'm not talking about cases of terminal illness and euthanasia.) It's not that he wouldn't let me do it, it's not that he wouldn't hold still for it, it's that I believe that it would be a terrible waste, and I would get in serious trouble karmically for that. Not to mention the death-in-prison thing afterwards, and being utterly heartbroken, and having ruined two lives.

And yes, some people do make their livestock into pets—but then they're pets, not really livestock any more. The other small farmers and homesteaders with whom I deal understand the difference—we sigh and say, "The kids have fallen in love with that turkey, and now it's a pet, and that means we can't kill and eat it, we have to let it die of old age. Bah." Calling something livestock presupposes a certain amount of emotional distance, at least as I understand the definition, and as I experience the reality of it. I've not personally made any of my livestock animals into my pets, but other folk attached to this farm have, and would be terribly upset to have to shoot them.

To each their own definition ... but living close to it, I can say that for me there is a great emotional distance between something that you could—if sadly—shoot, cook and eat, or at least shoot and calmly burn or bury, and something that (assuming you hadn't gone off the deep end) it would screw with you pretty seriously to have to kill off and dispose of. (And if it *wouldn't* screw with you emotionally to kill your slave, I personally am unsure as to whether you ought to own one. Call me conservative on that bit.)

I think that this idea romanticizes the idea of "livestock" in the minds of people who don't actually have any. Maybe it's fun and sexy to characterize your slave as a broodsow or whatever ... but the reality is different. The reality is knowing that if they don't breed, there's no milk or replacements or meat supply, and if they do breed, there is going to be surplus that has to go into the freezer. Even beloved Daisy the milk cow had to be forcibly bred every year until her death in order to get that milk, and what do you think happened to her calf? Especially if it was male.

I'm not saying that you can't play games with the idea. Sure, put your slave in ears and a tail and stick them in the barn, and pretend they're livestock. Go for it. call them a broodsow, or a milk cow, or a stud, or a prize gelding, if it turns you both on. But it's just a game, because it is not about life and death.

Q: My master just blew up and hit me in anger. It scared me. We've been together for years and he's never done anything like this. I don't know if I can trust him now.

Raven: My first thought is: How much stress is this man under, and does he have an outlet for it? People who are normally under tight control who suddenly lose it, well, they didn't just get there out of nowhere. One has to have a regular place to vent, to relax, maybe to lose it in a safe space and a safe way for an hour or two. And I mean *regular*, not a once-a-year vacation. If you don't let off the steam in little bits, it will eventually explode.

What makes things worse for slave-owners is that some feel that they can't let their slave be that outlet. Perhaps seeing the owner fall apart for an hour, even in a safe way, even if they then get back up and in the saddle again, will undermine the slave's need to see them as always in control, every minute of every day. Perhaps the owner only *thinks* that the slave feels this way. Either way, this can make for a difficult situation, especially if the slave is also the primary partner and the owner is a reclusive type. Performance anxiety is a big silent problem for masters, considering how constantly scrutinized we are by our slaves.

Does he have a safe space to periodically meltdown, or at least vent, including being able to vent about you and the enslavement process? Friends to talk to? A journal? A therapist? Something? It sounds to me like he had just bottled up all the stress of constant mastery—and you have no idea how stressful that can be, especially if your own life is having difficulty—until it boiled over. We are all human, and we all need outlets for our stress. I have learned this the hard way. Maybe finding him some stress-venting outlet would be a way in which you could help him out?

In the meantime, you should express to him that your trust in his self-control is in danger of being damaged, and you have the right to expect an answer that takes your feelings seriously, and tells you what he intends to do to make sure that the problem does not continue.

Q: How can you be happy with a vanilla relationship along with your slave? Aren't you a dominant? Wouldn't you automatically prefer a slave?

Raven: Well, I have an egalitarian wife and a slaveboy, and I don't think that anyone who knows me personally would say that I'm not an alpha. But people love people for all sorts of reasons. People fall in love across all sorts of boundaries that they never thought they'd cross—"Oh, gods, not one of *them!* How do I have a relationship with one of *them!*" And, sometimes, with time and work and compromise, and enough love, it can all work out.

I love my wife very much. We have been together for 16 years and we have no intention of leaving each other. We are also both very strong-willed and aggressive people, and she has no intention of being submissive to me—nor would it be fair of me to ask that of her when it's not in her nature. Yet I am an alpha, very much a dominant. So how do we work this thing?

Well, let's start with the fact that I'm not a slave to my own dominance. What I mean by that is that I am not uncontrollably overbearing to everyone else in the world, including everyone who didn't sign up for that (which would be everyone except Joshua). I do not crack a whip at the waitress, nor shout orders at the cashier. I do not tell my friends where to work or who to have sex with. I don't tell other submissives that they ought to treat me special just because I happen to own someone who isn't them. In other words, I have self-control, and I can restrict dominant *behavior* to appropriate places.

Would I rather have my wife be submissive to me? Actually, I'd rather have *everyone* be submissive to me, in my fantasies. I'd love to be King of the World, but that isn't gonna happen. And I'm OK with that. It would be immature not to be. If I was so enslaved to my own dominance that I couldn't have any close relationships unless I was in charge, I'd have no friends. (Actually, I've met quite a few self-proclaimed domly-doms who seem to have no friends. Is that the mark of a "real" dominant—someone who is so stuck on constantly being one-up on everyone that they are incapable of doing otherwise? Seems like a handicap to me. Rather have friends, thanks.)

My wife is one more person in the world who isn't going to kowtow to me, and because I love her, that isn't necessary. If she were submissive, she'd be a different person, not the person that I know and love. I like her fire and spirit and willfulness. It can be fun to watch. I have learned, over time, not to aim my dominance at her. And there are things she wants that I can't give her—a partner who isn't chronically ill, for example. It's not perfect, but there's a lot of love between us, and we've made it work so far.

On the other hand, I do better with a place to put it, or it will leak out—not only onto her, but onto everyone else as well. We are all three polyamorous—and wouldn't be together if we weren't—so I get from Joshua what I can't get from her, or from anyone else in the world for that matter. It works.

I hope that's an example of how such a situation can work out. Fortunately for me I am poly by nature and am not so restricted in my choices.

Q: How would you feel about losing your slave?

Raven: When I lost my first slave, it was like there was a big hole in me … that I didn't know had been there until it had slowly been filled with the willing submission of another human being, and then was suddenly ripped empty again. The wind blew through it. I was desolate.

Skip forward some years, a few short-lived subs, and then I get another one. I made the mistake of falling in love, again. This boy left me after a year and a half, because I was moving away and the boy didn't want to follow—it would have been havoc to school and career. Besides, there were serious religious differences that were causing problems. This time I was ready for it, but it still hurt for about a year.

When I finally found the right boy (some years and short-lived subs later), I had given up on ownership. It was too much emotion to sink into something that could up and leave, and rip a big piece of your heart out. It's not just about love. Ownership, for me, has emotions all its own that are, in many ways, more intense than love, and almost indescribable. We don't have the words for them. Anyhow, Joshua practically had to cajole me into believing in it again.

The Property: Attitude and Surrender

Q: What do you get out of being a slave, anyway, Joshua?

Joshua: Primarily, I get the opportunity to do something real and meaningful with my life. While I wasn't exactly discontented with my life prior to being owned, it had never occurred to me to expect any kind of deep fulfillment or purpose from life. Now that I have that, I would not want to be without it. By my actions in service I am able to contribute to greater goals, rather than just keeping myself fed and housed and entertained.

It gives me purpose. My master is doing great work in the world, and by serving him I support that work. I can do more good for the world by serving him than I could on my own. There is a quote I like very much, "There are two ways of spreading light—being the candle or the mirror that reflects it." I am the mirror, and that's valuable work too.

Slavery is remarkably intimate. I never would have tolerated a relationship this intimate without a power dynamic. I prefer to keep people at a distance, and Raven doesn't permit that. Having this level of intimacy is challenging, but immensely rewarding.

It prompts spiritual growth. It is an intense and demanding relationship that brings up a lot of issues. Raven tends to force me to work on these issues even when I'd choose to ignore them and run away. In theory I could do as much work on myself all on my own, but in this relationship, I can't avoid it. I'm not a hugely self-disciplined person, so this is good.

It creates an obligation to take care of myself. Raven doesn't want me damaging his property by eating unhealthily, driving recklessly, using recreational drugs, not getting enough sleep, or doing any of the countless things which are bad for me but in the past I often decided were "worth it". He can require that I act in my own long-term best interest, because he doesn't place a high value on me gratifying my fleeting desires.

It makes me accountable. My behavior reflects on Raven, and that holds me to a higher standard of behavior than I'd otherwise be inclined to keep. I can be fairly, um, ethically flexible when left to my own devices.

It teaches me how to spiritually surrender my ego. It is easier for me to surrender to a person in a very tangible way than to surrender myself to the All-That-Is, but the tangible sort of surrender is very good training for the higher sort of surrender. That may be a bit esoteric, but it is a primary motivation for me.

I also get to bring comfort and happiness to someone who I love passionately and deeply. I have deep trust and radical honesty with someone who knows and understands everything about me, and loves me exactly as I am. I get the best sex I've ever had.

I love my job.

Q: We're attempting a Master/slave relationship, but I'm really struggling with the things that are asked of me. I'm supposed to do my duty as a slave, not just willingly, but happily. How do I do this when it's something I hate? My feelings are my feelings.

Raven: First, this is as much your master's responsibility as your own. If he's inexperienced, he may have little idea how to hold up his end of it, which is indeed something not so easy. But ... let's break things down.

The biggest part of any slave's job is attitude adjustment. Learning how to adjust your attitude is probably the most important and valuable skill that any slave can learn. That's something that Joshua stresses to all the novices who email him and ask, "What do I have to learn in order to be a good slave?" He tells them to practice learning to like things that they wouldn't normally like. Any things. Toy trains. Buffy the

Vampire Slayer. Girl Scout Cookies. Anal sex. Golden showers. Ironing. Whatever. The more and different things that you are able to apply this skill to, the better.

So you, as the slave, have a responsibility to learn how to do this thing. Luckily, it sounds like you have plenty of dislikes to apply it to. Luckily, because this skill may take years to master. However … you don't do this in a vacuum. Well, if you're really experienced at it, you can. But you sound like you and your master are just starting out with this stuff, and you can't be expected to just change your attitude and feelings towards any random painful thing on command, any more than you can be asked to flap your arms and fly, or stop having that headache or stubbed toe pain. It doesn't work that way, and your master needs to understand that. A mature person doesn't demand what is (at least currently) beyond the slave's ability to give, or at least if they ask for it, they shouldn't penalize the slave for not being able to come through on it.

And a wise master would rather have the slave express their displeasure than have them hide it behind a fake smile. Yes, pleasure would be better, but if you currently only have a choice between those two, pick the former. And, frankly, if you cannot emotionally bear to see your slave less than happy in any way, you are in the wrong business.

I'm not saying that an owner shouldn't care about the slave's feelings, nor be responsive to them in some way at least. But the "training" part of the job—and here I don't mean putting a slave through some fetishy paces, I mean slowly conditioning them to see things the owner's way, want the things that the owner values, and change in ways that personally serve the owner—requires that sometimes, the slave is going to be frustrated, or fail, or be discomfited. And who can they go to with that, and not be reprimanded or rejected for it, if not to the one in charge of the process?

It's the owner's job to acknowledge their trouble, give them positive reinforcement of whatever type they've established works on that slave, and help to figure out ways in which the slave can work towards liking the "whatever" better. If that sounds like a huge and complex and confusing job, that's because it is. And that's why owning a human being is not a job for just anyone.

If you are the sort of person who has a malleable personality (and, frankly, that's a serious benefit for a slave), the "fake it till you feel it" approach can really work well. If you're not that sort—if you're more the rigid control freak type—then it probably won't work. (Sure as heck doesn't work worth a damn for me.) If the s-type wants to try this, the best thing to do is to go to the owner and say, "Hey, I want to try this fake-it-till-you-feel-it thing on this activity that I hate and you want me to like. I don't know if it'll work, but it's worth a shot. So I'd like to try pretending to like it the next few times you do it, in the hopes that it will work. That means that there will be a bit of faking going on, but since you know that I'm doing it and why, it's not dishonesty. I will keep you posted as to whether it's working, and if it doesn't work after (X many agreed-upon number of) times, I will tell you and we'll try something else." This has worked for Joshua many times.

If that approach doesn't work, another approach is to concentrate on how much this pleases your owner, and/or taking pride in doing the job well in spite of how much you hate it, and/or how it reinforces your slavery to know that you must do this thing you don't like. Any of these can be lifeboats in the storm, something to hold onto to get you through the hard parts.

Q: My boyfriend is my first dominant, and we're both new to this. I'm supposed to go with him and be OK with the things he wants to do, and usually I'm all right with that. But he isn't willing to go with me and take part in the things I want to do, ever, and once in a while I'd like it to be my turn to pick our activities! It makes me feel isolated, and like my creativity is

being stifled, like who I am is draining away. Is a master obligated in any way to give a little mutuality?

Raven: Joshua and I have somewhat different answers to this question. Egalitarian couples generally trade off with such things, even if they aren't always that enjoyable to both parties, because the idea is that if I go to your boring tennis match, you'll come to my (similarly boring in your eyes) art museum. We try to be as good about it as we can, because we love each other and want to see the other one happy, and because we want them to respond similarly.

A Master/slave demographic is different. The Master or Mistress has no obligation to humor the slave. If that's done at all, it's done out of a sense of generosity and mercy, and the slave should not get to the point of feeling entitled to it. If an owner is keeping their property locked up to the point where isolation is affecting their mental health, it's probably wise for them to allow the slave to go out and have a social life. But no one's mental health was ever compromised because their partner wouldn't go with them to the tennis match. In fact, it's good for the slave's mental health to have solo activities that they enjoy and friends who share their interests, because it teaches them not to be dependent on the dominant for every scrap of fulfillment.

On the other hand, if it makes you unhappy to be in a relationship that doesn't have any of those egalitarian-style obligations, there's no reason to go that far down the D/s spectrum. The level of power dynamic in a relationship must be what is comfortable for both people involved. You and your partner need to figure out what percentage of your interactions will be D/s, and which will be egalitarian. You need to defend your boundaries in this matter, and not go further than you're comfortable with. If you need part of the relationship to be egalitarian enough that he is obligated to go with you to your friends' house or your tennis game or whatever, that needs to be negotiated. You have the right to say, "We go this far down that road, but no further. I am only submissive to you to this extent." He has no right to push you further than that. If it's gone beyond where you're comfortable, back up.

Joshua: First of all, it is possible for many submissives to genuinely adapt to their dominant's interests. I don't mean that they learn to put up with them, or learn to take some satisfaction in their dominant's enjoyment of them. I mean that they sincerely come to enjoy the activities their dominant enjoys, regardless of whether their dominant is currently involved in it. This can also mean that the activities they were once very interested in that the dominant dislikes can become less important to them. These types of relationships have a way of shifting the submissive's internal priorities to match the dominant. So if you are malleable and work on internalizing the dominant's preferences, this doesn't need to be a hardship in the long term.

Secondly, I worry about submissives who only seem to be happy when their dominant is with them and paying attention to them. If you have independent interests that are important to you, it shouldn't matter whether your dominant is interested in doing them with you. Talk with your dominant about setting aside a reasonable amount of time and resources for you to enjoy these activities, and then go have fun. If you don't already have friends who share your interests, try to make some. Don't let this relationship isolate you.

Lastly, on an esoteric level, I find it important to remember that my core self is not about what activities I enjoy or who I socialize with. You can't lose who you are by abandoning some hobbies. One of the great challenges of deep submission (and one of its great benefits) is in learning to find that core self that exists when all of the superficial aspects of identity are stripped away. Deep submission teaches you how to sacrifice the ego, the "I am", as well as the "I want", the "I have", the "I like", and the "I do". Don't ignore or bury any uncomfortable feelings you have about what activities you and your dominant engage in, but this might help to try putting the issue in a larger perspective.

Q: What happens when the slave gets so good at the job that it's easy, and they aren't challenged any more? Does the dominant have to come up with more and greater tasks for them to do, so that they can feel enslaved?

Raven: OK ... let me get this straight and make sure that I understand you. We're talking about a slave who measures their level of enslavement by their level of discomfort and suffering?

I can see that if a submissive has been dealing with a dominant who continually defaults to the slave's wishes in obvious ways, so that the slave feels like they're not really being mastered but just humored, there might be some reactive behavior around that. But as long as the dominant is actually using the submissive—emphasis on using—in order to achieve the dominant's goals, and the dominant is contented with their performance, then the slave should get over it.

If the slave's complaint is that they aren't feeling enslaved enough, the dominant trying harder to please and humor them by inconveniencing him/herself further is not the way to solve the problem. I've never personally dealt with a slave who required that kind of confirmation. If I did, I think that it would be one of the things about them that I would endeavor to change.

Which is the real challenge, if you want challenges. Instead of looking at it from the point of view of "My slave has this annoying emotional need that possibly comes from some kind of past damage, and it means that I have to adjust all my orders or requirements or expectations in order to not set them off," look at it from the point of view of: "My slave has this annoying emotional reaction that cramps my style. Can we change that? Let's make it a long-term goal to change that."

How about this for an exchange?

Slave: I don't feel challenged enough. Everything I'm doing has become comfortable and boring. It's too easy. I don't feel like a real slave, being made to do painful things.

Owner: Look, I'm in charge here, and what I say goes. And I want a slave who is happy and content with their lot, even if that lot is just to do the same hundred services for me for the rest of their life. So if you want a challenge, how about getting rid of that attitude you just spouted, and taking on a new attitude of being content with whatever you're given? How's that for a challenge? That ought to keep you busy for a while.

Scary, eh? (Said with a big grin.)

Q: How does a slave get over their attachment to the M/s ideal in their head? Or should they? Maybe they should just find someone who matches it perfectly?

Joshua: They had better, or it will prevent them from fully submitting, even if their M-type has similar ideals. Of course, that's easier said than done. For the first year or so, I had very firm ideas of what sort of acts of dominance Raven ought to be doing. At the time we were both feeling things out with our relationship. I had a somewhat clearer idea of how this sort of thing worked because I didn't have years and years of experience in the play BDSM scene and the feminist non-violence movement and all that, like he did. So, slavey or not, we had a long period where I could legitimately say "No, no, this is the way things are supposed to go," because I could see that he was acting from his past relationship baggage rather than from his own will. Eventually, though, he got through 95% of that baggage, and my insight into the "correct way" for these things to go became more of a hindrance than a help.

But I was still in the habit, so I kept at it. I was going through a difficult time in my life for unrelated reasons, and I unfairly blamed a lot of it on my master being insufficiently dominant with me. There were things that many masters do—like set strict hour-by-hour schedules—that I very much wanted to have and he was not at all interested in providing. He'd try it out, but it was just to humor me and it never lasted.

Eventually when I was bitching and moaning about this one night he dragged me outside into the sheep pasture and gave me a formal reprimand for it. He's only done that one or two other times in our relationship, so it had serious impact. He told me that there would be no more complaining about this—he would exert his authority over me in the way he chose to, not the way I wanted him to. It took a number of months for that to really sink in, but it did. I think that the first step is the owner really knowing and communicating what he wants and why, and the second step is the slave getting over themselves. See the question on Being Right for more about that.

Q: How do you get your owner to give you appreciation when you need it?

Joshua: My master thanks me as he pleases. He says that one of the reasons he enjoys being around me is that he doesn't have to mind what he says or does for my benefit.

I enjoy it when the things I do obviously delight my master, but I like anything that delights him, no matter who did it. If his enjoyment of the thing was the whole point of me doing it, then if he doesn't give me any indication that he enjoyed it, I'll tend to wonder if I've done it well enough. I don't get resentful without that acknowledgment, but I do tend to get insecure.

He has taught me to ask him flatly for an assessment of my work and take it at face value regardless of the tone it is issued in. If he says something like "It's fine, now get on with your work," that is enough. Under no circumstances am I to decide he didn't really like it because he "sounded upset with me" or "didn't act appreciative". If he is brooding I am supposed to remember that even though I spend a lot of my time thinking about him, he doesn't spend nearly as much time thinking about me, so I shouldn't take his moods personally. If I feel like I need a head pat, I'll say, "I'd like a head pat, sir." That's my way of asking for any form of appreciation—I didn't intend for it to be literal, but sometimes he's given me literal pats on the head. Whether or not he gives it to me has almost nothing to do with the quality of my service.

In other words, if you know that you're going to need a certain amount of appreciation, make sure that your dominant is understanding about that, and ask them to come up with useful and reasonably convenient ways and times for you to ask for it. If you stand around and wait for it to appear, you might be waiting a long time.

Q: What happens when the slave needs attention and the owner needs time alone? How do you balance that?

Raven: It is not always easy. I suppose that for me, since I've been the single parent of a high-need learning-disabled child (now grown and flown), I spent 18 years being conditioned to put down the work and tend to the annoying human responsibility with as much grace as I could muster, and curbing my irritation because I know it's better to deal with a small explosion now than a terrible one later. After my daughter, who required homeschooling for her entire childhood, Joshua is easy. He's a reasonably self-sufficient and introspective adult. (This will probably make people wince, but like I said in the first chapter, you'd be surprised how many skills carry over nicely from parenting to M/s. Just because the parent's job is to provide a safe and happy atmosphere for the child doesn't mean that the kid doesn't know which of them is in charge.)

I'm fairly self-sufficient and can happily spend hours and even days alone without a problem, as long as I have interesting work to do. Indeed, I often get obsessive about my work, and this means that Joshua doesn't get as much time and attention from me as he'd like. I know that he gets lonely sometimes, and I encourage him to come and tell me when it happens. Sometimes I am so busy that I have to send him away again, but usually I can do something, even let him curl up around me while I read or do other work. Physical contact helps him a lot. I expect some of the separation anxicty is due to the enslavement—as he's put it in autistic-spectrum terms, he "orients" to me, which is why he can't concentrate on writing anything when I'm standing over him.

Being ignored for long periods of time is very difficult for him. I know that it helps him when I give him specific things to do with that time, with orders to check in periodically, rather than just leaving him to his own devices. Sometimes I get caught up in work and end up ignoring him anyway, though. That's life with an obsessed owner.

I think that the biggest problem is "skin hunger". Most slaves have to adapt to having their bodily space constantly violated by their owner, at a moment's notice. Their flesh is not their own, and that physical boundary of body autonomy doesn't exist between them and their owner. (And yes, that's one of the tools used to create enslavement.) Unlike a situation where someone is repeatedly violated without prior consent by the touch of people they don't trust—which leads to dissociation from the body—since they have initially consented and do (ideally) trust the owner, they simply adjust to it and (usually) find it a source of comfort, or at least "the way it's supposed to be". Adjusting positively to constant physical violation from a trusted, comforting source means that they can get to need it, and feel weird when hours or days go by without it. So I can understand how "skin hunger" can be much worse for an owned slave of many years. I'd expect that it might even change their heads to the point where their mind is screaming for alone time but their body is screaming for touch. Perhaps it could be resolved by curling up together to watch a movie or read without actual interaction.

On the other hand, there's the problem of attention, and whose needs are more critical. There was a point in the past where Joshua became ill for a significant period of time, on top of me with my chronic illness. It wasn't his fault, but he sucked up a great deal of time and attention that would have otherwise been put into my work. The fact that my illness was progressing meant that there were quite a few times when I desperately needed to be the one on the receiving end of help, but he was in a bad way, so he got the time and attention. Why? Because I had sworn to be the one in charge, and that means that the responsibility was mine. Not his to decide, but mine. And, also, I was and am stronger than he is. Not that he's a total weakling, but when it comes to willpower I am stronger than 90% of the people I know. So I could bear it better than he could. It wasn't entitlement, it was mercy.

I think that the fact that I do not do the reward/punishment thing helped him with seeing it as mercy. As he's commented elsewhere, when he screws up I show my disappointment in him (which is really all it takes to make him feel completely awful and penitent), and we discuss how to make sure this doesn't happen again; conversely, if he does something right, maybe I notice and comment, maybe I don't. I try to remember to compliment him periodically, and I do nice things for him, but they are not rewards. They are whims, generosity, mercy. Knowing that this is why he gets anything extra from me—I've made a decision to be generous for whatever reason of my own—helped with not seeing it as entitlement.

Joshua: I have to say that this was a really hard process for me. I'm still working on it, but I have come a long way. I do encourage him to express his dominance over me in whatever way he pleases, because it is good for both of us. I just have to suggest it in a fun sexy way, not a whiny malcontented way. If he doesn't feel pressured to do it, he really enjoys it. When he's too busy or distracted to pay any attention to me at all, some days I can do fine, but some days I'm no good at feeling all submissive about it; my need for attention is actually greater than my need for acts of dominance. What I try to do is find things that are the most emotionally satisfying for me while being the least annoying to him. So long as I get some kind of physical contact I'm usually okay, so I'll be proactive about it and go snuggle up to him while he talks on the phone. He may still ignore me, but being ignored when I'm right there is actually pretty emotionally satisfying. Being actively ignored in the other room is not.

Also, when I'm doing a lot of unsupervised outside work, it really helps when he praises me for it in a way that affirms that these are things I am doing in service to him. It is particularly good when he makes it clear that he does have a standard for my outside behavior, that he is paying some attention to what I'm doing, and that he is pleased to see that I am meeting his standards without creating more work for him.

The absolute hardest thing is spending my time doing things away from him that he doesn't seem to give a damn about. I try hard to remember that he cares deeply about the big-picture goals, even if he doesn't want to hear me natter on about every detail, but it is tough. It is easy to be self-motivating when he shows enthusiasm for my day-to-day activities, but no matter how much he wants me to get my degree, he isn't going to show enthusiasm for the orthopedic assessment and treatment of stenosing tenosynovitis. I have to rely on my own resources to carry me through, and that can be scary and lonely.

It helps that I have a strong sense of spiritual meaning in my life that isn't entirely dependent on my service to Raven. I feel like the outside work I do has inherent value, so even if Raven is more indifferent than I'd like about my work, I can take satisfaction in that.

Q: We're just starting out in M/s, and my master works late and often gets home tired. I want his attention, but he sometimes sends me away because he's too tired to master me, and it hurts so much! I can't bear it. The words "I need some

time away from you to decompress," even if they're honest, are terribly hurtful. How do I cope?

Raven: Those are only hurtful words if you've decided that they are.

That's what we're talking about when we say that attitude adjustment is a slave's best tool. Could you become the sort of person for whom those words wouldn't be hurtful? Could you become the sort of person who, if your master said those words to you, would automatically take them as no more than "He's in a bad way, he's tired, is there something I can do to help him that asks nothing of him? Is the best thing I can do to go away and give him space? If so, I'll do it and be glad that there is something I can do..."? Could you become the sort of person who could hear those words and never take it personally?

What would it take for you to become that person? Look down that road, even a little, even if it hurts, even if it seems impossible. What would it take to be that person?

And now you're thinking, but that's all on me, and it seems like such a big task to change myself! Isn't the master supposed to be taking responsibility here? And yes, you're right. Here the master's job comes in. It is to *admit that this kind of person is the kind of slave that would work best for them*, and to figure out how to help you achieve that.

His job is not to spare you that thing, but to help make you into the sort of person for whom it wouldn't be a problem. Read that again, until you understand it thoroughly. I will not bore you with how many times I have gone down that road—wanting to spare my slave rather than go to the trouble of changing him. The first trouble is even admitting that this thing, this situation which might make my slave want to weep and run, is really what I'd prefer, given my way. The second trouble is figuring out how to help them change. Those might seem insurmountable to an inexperienced master—especially a tired and overworked one.

(Yes, you do have to spare a slave if you've tried everything and they absolutely can't change. You have to work with what you've got. But people are a lot more flexible than they'd believe ... and, frankly, if you're not flexible, being a slave will be very hard for you.)

So start with that thought. Every time that your master does something that upsets you, ask yourself: Could I be someone for whom this is not a problem? What would it take to make me that person? Maybe you'll be able to see your way down that road, maybe not. Either way, bring it to him (not when he's staring blearily into space, but later) and share this struggle, and ask for help. Maybe have some ideas ready as to what might help, at least on the ones where you have some idea what it might take.

And know this is a process that grows slowly over time. The more you do this successfully, the easier it will become. Change in small ways, ways that you can see your way to, and the bigger ways will become easier. You'll be slowly learning—with the help of your master—to become adaptable, and adaptability is the single most important attribute of any slave, period. And simultaneously, your master will learn better how to help you with it, by observation of how you work and what works to change you. Each success will teach him, too. Eventually, he may take over entirely, and you'll just be changed and won't notice it. But he won't get there overnight, and that path takes practice, and many small successes that can be observed. You need to get really, really invested in giving him those successes.

Start small. Start with that little thing ... those words. See where you can go.

As for the immediate problem of your master being too tired to master you: If you live together—and you're a reasonably service-oriented slave, not a needy prince/ss—and you have a close relationship, then it's easier for the owner to say, "Look, I'm overwhelmed right now. The service I need you to perform today (or this week) is to be self-sufficient enough not to need my direction, and to do items XYZ which will help lighten my load and help me recover." Maybe that's taking on extra work, maybe that's physical comfort, maybe that's just taking a break from *explicit* slaveyness (although it is always *implicit*, you're doing this on orders) and being a supportive companion for a while. If you're the slave, and you're right there seeing your owner struggle, helping them get their wheels back under them will be more important to you at that moment than your own need to be "managed"—and ideally it will be done for their sake, not primarily so you can get back to being comfortably managed.

Q: What if the slave is Right?

Joshua: One of the things that a slave needs to get over is the dependence on seeing themselves as Right, and knowing that other people hear their opinions and agree. I think it is easier for some people to simply be routinely denied the opportunity to express any opinion than to have their opinion asked and either taken or disregarded as the master chooses. There is a pervasive idea in many people that if you communicate your ideas clearly to someone, and they really listen and are open to hearing you, then obviously they will do what you want. (Because you are so obviously right!) If they don't, then either they are just stubborn, or don't respect you, or don't value your opinion, or you need to explain it better.

Also, for a *lot* of folks, being right is one of the most important things in the world. It's more important even than getting their way. Many folks would rather be told, "You are right, but I'm still not giving you what you want," than, "You are wrong, but I'll give you what you want anyway."

Slaves have to get over that, because in the end it doesn't matter if they think that they are right. Either they trust the judgment of the person to whom they have given themselves, or they don't. (And if they don't, why are they enslaved to them?) There are going to be a lot of situations where the slave is going to get vetoed, and that's what they signed up for. Asking someone else to be In Charge means that you do what they say, even if you think that brand of dishwashing detergent won't do as sparkling a job as this one. Usually, it is better to just be obedient in trivial situations. Letting go of needing to be right will save your sanity in the end.

My master says he'd rather be right than look right, so if the matter is of any importance, he expects me to tell him when I think he is mistaken about something or has overlooked something. But if he disagrees and it isn't relevant to any major decision-making, I try to fall back on saying something like, "Well, you know my opinion on such things," after the first protest, and then drop it.

If it was something important, I'd offer whatever supporting evidence I could, but repeating myself or getting upset doesn't convince him of anything. Besides, the ideal goal isn't to prove that I am right. It is to present the information I have to him so he can make an accurate assessment of the situation. I try to think of it in terms of information, not argument. I give him the information, and he comes to whatever conclusion he comes to.

If I am really upset about it, I'll tell him. That is information too, but it is only information the first time I say it. Maybe a second time if I think he is seriously underestimating how upset I am. Beyond that, I'm just whining. And truthfully, I'm not very good at this. I tend to be whiny. I am working on it, and working on recognizing the line between what is real information, what is leading comments, and what is thinly veiled criticism. (The blatant criticism I know is out of line, but I still do it when I get riled up.) The more I work on this issue the more I notice when other people do it, and it makes me uncomfortable. It gets me thinking how annoying and obvious it is, and how I'm likely just as annoying and obvious when I do it.

And isn't the idea that people can get by just fine without our advice so humbling? That our opinion would be of little enough benefit to them that they can safely disregard it? That they can make their own decisions entirely without our input? Terrible thought!

Q: My master made me so angry today that after trying three times to tell him that he was pissing me off, and having him ignore it, I screamed at him—and then when I told him that he'd ruined my morning, he said that I'd allowed my morning to be ruined!

Raven: He's right.

A slave's single biggest task is attitude adjustment. Period. Ideally, you should be constantly striving to find a better attitude about things asked of you that are difficult, and that includes putting up with your master's bad moods, maybe being asked to absorb some of that and not take it personally, maybe being the one place in the whole world where he can let his hair down and not watch what he says all the bloody time, and not get in trouble for it.

You perhaps have no idea what kind of an amazing service that is for someone who has strong, unacceptable emotions but has to watch themselves around others. To know that I can just say whatever I want around Joshua, that he knows me well enough to not take personally what shouldn't be taken personally, that he is good enough at attitude adjustment (usually, he sometimes has his bad days too) to roll with the punches and put up with behaviors of mine that annoy him without asking me to be careful around him ... that's amazing. In other words, with him I can really relax. You have no idea how wonderful it is to be with someone who isn't going to react oversensitively to your genuine expression of emotion.

I don't know either you or your master, nor what your dynamic is like, so any advice I give might be useless. However, I would say that if it were me, and my slave was trying to let me know that I was upsetting them, and I didn't get the message ... once we'd talked it out later, I'd find them ways of telling me such things that would get my attention, and perhaps gain my sympathy. For example, snarling at me is not going to make me want to immediately back off from whatever I'm doing and stop upsetting them. Someone I didn't own, sure. But not my slave. Instead, I might tell them: If I'm upsetting you, plead with me to stop. Say, "Please, sir, what you're saying/doing is really hurting me. I know it's your right to say/do it, but please, please could you stop?"

By this, the slave is acknowledging the following:

a) that they are hurt and upset,

b) that they acknowledge that I have the right to hurt and upset them in this way (we're assuming that this is something not explicitly negotiated that the M-type has given their word, for whatever reason, not to do),

c) that they acknowledge that they have no right to expect me to stop,

d) that what they are asking for is not justice but mercy. This makes me a lot more likely to be merciful.

The next thing that you can do is that you can step back from the behavior, and ask yourself, "In the grand scheme of things, is this really all that huge a deal?" You assume that it will happen again, and you work on ways to not be caught off guard, so that when it does happen again (or something like it) you can shrug it off. "That's just the way he is, and it pleases him to have me just accept him the way he is, without his having to change for me. And really, in the big picture, it's not such a big deal."

If you really think that his behavior is dishonorable or unethical, of course, that's a different problem, and you will have to ask him to change, or you'll leave. But be very clear what your standards are, and whether this is a matter of ethics or mere discomfort.

Q: When my master gives me treats, I feel terrible. Especially when they're not on the diet he set for me. I feel guilty, even though it's his order. Is this bad?

Raven: That, and it's rejecting a gift of mercy.

Joshua isn't allowed to eat sugar. If I bend on that and mercifully give him one bite of my ice cream—not because he's been especially good, but because I am feeling generous at the moment—that's not just because it's slave-maintenance. I enjoy being able to give him the occasional gift and see him smile. For him to refuse my gift out of some need for martyrdom, that isn't what I want. Ideally, he should be able to ask for a bite of my ice cream, and if it's No, accept gracefully and without resentment, and if it's Yes, accept gratefully and with joy.

So, really, what's more important in your mind here: your owner's wish to give you a gift, or your own need to feel as if you are in control of your diet (which you aren't)?

Joshua: I would characterize this as "mercy" rather than "inconsistency". When I've seen inconsistency in a power dynamic it has been where the top acts arbitrarily, pampering and punishing at their whim rather than in direct response to anything the slave does. It is the opposite of many kinds of training.

I do think that mercy is an enforcer of power, when given sparingly. However, if there is a sense in the slave that the master's mercy can be appealed to or counted on, then it can tend to encourage emotional manipulation by the slave. If the master loves the slave, this is extremely likely. It can also serve to reward the display of suffering, and encourage a certain sort of martyrdom. On the other hand, receiving the occasional unlooked-for mercy can be a wonderful thing that increases the slave's sense of devotion, and reinforces that comforting as well as difficult things come from the owner's hand.

If this is happening frequently enough that you think that he's sabotaging his own goal, ask him what his priorities are in this situation. If he isn't rigidly invested in the diet, that's one thing. Submissives are by nature inclined to martyrdom, and he may have your best interests in mind. Either way, it's appropriate for you to ask him to clarify his position.

Q: What's the hardest thing for a submissive to give up?

Raven: That depends on the slave in question, and their values. But one of the hardest things to give up, I think, is control over your "look". In Western society, we use our look to communicate a lot of our individualism, and to have that taken away is difficult. Ask anyone who's gone into the military or joined a convent/monastery/ashram. Slaves often have a rough time of it when suddenly they realize that they have to keep their hair, clothing, and body presenting the appearance that the owner wants to the world, even if that's not how they've been thinking of themselves. A lot of reactance battles are fought over bluejeans and shades of lipstick, not to mention haircuts.

We're taught, all our lives, that it's important to express one's self publicly, ideally through look and presentation and demeanor. To have an owner yank that around to something different can feel artificial, and possibly stifling. To have an owner change that out from under you while you aren't looking can be a shock when it catches up to you.

When I got Joshua, he looked like a typical punk kid—mohawk, septum piercing, earplugs, ripped jeans with obscene slogans on them. He looked that way because his roommates looked that way, and he felt that he might as well copy them. I changed that—not all at once, but slowly.

His friends noticed—they sent him a homemade going-away card when he left to live with me, and it had cartoons illustrating the differences between "Old Josh" and "New Josh" on it, which I think was their way of processing the situation. At least "New Josh" had a smile, while "Old Josh" was sullen.

One day after we'd been together for about a year, and we were at a conference, he woke me up and told me that he'd just looked in the mirror and it hit him like a ton of bricks. There he was, his hair and beard grown out, septum ring gone (it interfered with vigorous oral sex), ears back to normal, dressed and groomed and acting like a Victorian manservant ... and he had to just stand there and stare and say, "What the hell happened to you?"

This was not a "look", an identity, he ever expected. I think he'd expected to be some biker leather daddy's pierced-up punk boy. (Not that there's anything wrong with that. It's just not me.) And at first it was just me making slow change after slow change, escalating, and him wanting to please me, and then, bam, he's staring at someone else in the mirror.

He was a bit stunned for a while. I remember a tearful question, later, of "Please tell me again that you wanted me this way!" But then he made peace with it, and it's been fine ever since. But I can understand the shock. I've been through it myself, with my religious activities, and with other things in my life. It can be unnerving, because "look" is a reflection of "me", and if "look" is different, then "me" must be different too, right? Maybe, maybe not, but in the case of a slave, probably yes.

(Joshua decided to answer this question as part of another one about Sacrifice in the *Religion and Spirituality* section.)

Q: How does a submissive learn their dominant's preferences, especially the ones that the dominant might not think to tell them?

Joshua: You watch them. Look at what they choose for themselves, and what things they seem to like or dislike. If you observe carefully, you'll probably be able to tell the difference between his genuine desires and him being gracious in public about something that might not be his first choice. If you are very emotionally invested in giving her what she wants (and you probably are), the more gracefully you can accept constructive criticism, the more comfortable a dominant may be with clarifying the more trivial aspects of their preferences. If you spend hours preparing a meal and then look at them with big pleading eyes while asking if everything was OK, you might not get the most useful feedback. On the other hand, if you grill them about every aspect of the meal—did he prefer butter to margarine, if the steak knife was sharp enough, if the beverage was too cold or too warm—they are likely to lose patience with you. You'll likely get more information from observing than from asking, but do ask occasionally to make sure that you're reading the signals correctly. I've found that when it comes to asking my master about preferences, it's been more useful to ask him whether he'd like to see something done again, rather than whether he thought that it was acceptable.

I'm also something of a perfectionist, and my internalization of his preferences means that I often obsess about how to do things his way ... but better than he'd ever think to want them done. The funniest thing about this is that masters rarely care about this level of detail. Sure, some trainer-types delight in giving a four-hour lesson on the proper way to make a bacon sandwich, but most aren't interested in what my master refers to as the "Which three eggs should I scramble, Master?" attitude. But sometimes, when getting food for my master, I pause at the silverware drawer and wonder which spoon I should get for him. I know my master's thought process about it would go something like, "Is it a spoon? Is it clean?" but I know that there are spoons I like better than other spoons. It is trivial, but there is a small preference there. Should I be sure to get my master the "best" spoon? But what are his criteria for determining the "best" spoon? Are they the same as mine?

After a while, though, you get the hang of it. Just like you know your own preferences well enough that you tend to pick your favorite bowl or spoon without thinking much about it, you get to know your master's preferences and it just comes naturally.

Q: What do you do with an intelligent, argumentative sub who has a lawyer's mind and is always looking for loopholes in orders and contracts?

Joshua: Weaseling my way around rules and finding loopholes comes very naturally to me, but it is never something I've dared to try with my master. I have a hard time imagining a D/s relationship where that level of disrespect would be even remotely acceptable.

I think what I would want to do with a lawyerly sub is draw up her "contract" in the worst parody of legalese I could manage. "...and by this contract, the party of the first part, slave joan, hereafter known as That Rotten Weasel, will hereby submit to..." Extra points for misspellings and flagrant misuse of legal jargon. Then I'd forbid her from making a single comment about any aspect of the contract to anyone, including me. Not one word. Just sign it.

That would amuse me terribly.

Raven: To answer seriously: First, I'd call them on it. I'd point out that this way of doing things is counterproductive to both our goals, and I'd go over those goals again. "Do you enjoy it when you gain some kind of control, when you gain the upper hand at least some of the time? Yes? Then maybe you should be looking at an egalitarian relationship. No? Then perhaps you should keep in mind what's really important here, and what's a hindrance." Then I'd emphasize the spirit of the law rather than the letter of it, and tell them that I am trusting them to understand that spirit, and follow it to the best of their ability even when they are unsure of the letter. I'd probably emphasize the trick of creating a small version of me in their head to refer to when I am not present: "What would my dominant want me to do in this situation?" That makes the rules-lawyering immaterial, and puts the basis for decisions where it belongs.

Q: Even though I'm owned, whenever a dominant speaks to me in that dominant voice, I swoon. I can't help it! How do I keep that for my owner?

Raven: I think that's one of the dangers of being a submissive at heart. Some people are just alphas, some people are exactly the opposite. Most are in the middle. But the natural s-types are vulnerable in that way to that feeling. Something instinctive in them just reacts to the presence of Dom-ness, in whatever form, unless it is overridden by great dislike, or anger, or the words of their actual dominant.

This used to happen a good deal to Joshua—he'd get all weak in the knees over dominant personality types, or even someone who wasn't that type but was temporarily doing "the dominant voice", as it were. Roommates took advantage of him. Anyone with the right attitude whom he liked even a little could have him sexually almost at any time for the asking. I did a lot of work on/with him, doing some voluntary mind-programming to convince his brain that this feeling would only be aimed at me, and that other dominants would merely make him feel respectful, but not in any way unable to defend his boundaries.

But the best way to keep a slave from being rolled by the dominant voice of another is to help them to internalize the fact that their submission, like their body, *is not theirs to give away any more.* It is about internalizing not just that "only my owner gets this reflex" but "this body, this will, this cooperation is my owner's property, and it is not mine to give away or even offer, and anyone who tries to take it is stealing something of my owner's, and I should react like I would if I found them pilfering from his suitcase." Their submission is the valuable property of their owner, and they are supposed to guard it for that owner. They have been delegated the authority to do so, as it resides physically with them, but that's all. Guard, not give out. That requires Good Boundaries. If you saw someone stealing your owner's wallet, would you just stand by? That sounds like an abstract thing that wouldn't help in the moment, but it *can* be internalized with the right work.

What sprang to my mind was a scene from the novel *Shogun*. The scene is set in medieval Japan, and a European sailor shipwrecked there has been taken on by the Shogun and assigned a wife and a mistress to help him navigate cultural waters. Local thugs want his pistols, plot to get them away from him, and tell him that he can't enter a particular building unless he leaves them outside. He gives them to his wife, and tells her to defend them with her life. She knows that she can't shoot the warriors who bully her and tell her to give them over, so she points them at herself and threatens to commit suicide right there—which will make them lose huge face and get in trouble with the Shogun. They back off, and she saves his guns.

I feel like this is how a slave who has been instructed to be submissive solely to one owner ought to feel about their submission. They should guard it with their life. They should be willing to sacrifice anything—including the joy that they get from going under for an attractive dominant—to protect their owner's property from others.

Joshua still hates confrontations, is unable to physically defend himself if attacked (he just gets a prey reaction and goes fetal), and will go a long way to avoid a fight, but he is now able to keep polite and respectful boundaries with other domly types effortlessly, with no emotional struggle.

Joshua: Certain kinds of "slave training" have the unfortunate side effects of making the slave A) more passive and less assertive in general, and B) less able to have and hold any boundaries at all, not just to the owner. This could be characterized as taking down all the slave's walls and throwing open all the doors. What my master did to me was more like going in and changing all the locks, and taking the key with him. It may be that the former version is more likely to happen with an inexperienced dominant, or one who isn't particularly possessive, or who eroticizes the slave being open to anyone and anything in some way. (Or maybe they *want* a slave who will be submissive to anyone.)

So if you have a slave who is too passive for her own good, who has lousy boundaries, how can you teach them otherwise? Especially if you're dealing with female slaves, they may never have had the chance to actually stand guard over something. They might have been raised to think that they are helpless, that they couldn't possibly stand up to someone, that guarding anything is a man's job. That means that they won't guard their own boundaries, and that's a problem, unless you intend to keep the girl locked in the house, and never allow her to leave or see anyone else unsupervised. Which, although it is the stuff of some people's fantasy, is a great minority in the M/s demographic.

So here are some suggestions for training exercises:

1) Have them go to a party, maybe even a vanilla one. Have the owner slap their wallet or some other item of value down on a public table, and tell the slave to stand there, don't let anyone touch it, and don't touch or move it unless someone looks like they are going to make a grab for it. I suppose one could send over an unknown volunteer or two to say, "Wow, someone left their wallet! I'll just take it to the Lost and Found..."

2) Go to a play party with a willing female volunteer. Strip her and tie her up, and put the other slave in charge of protecting her, telling her, "Don't let any strangers touch her." Then leave for an hour. (It would be good to have a couple of unknown protectors around in case she screws up.) This may be a better example than the wallet, because she will likely have more empathy with another submissive female in a

helpless position. You'd have to pick the right party—wild enough that some people might well approach and show interest, but not so wild that anyone gets forcibly manhandled or that violence might happen.

This is meant to be an object lesson: "See that? That's your submissive nature. That's how you're to treat it when others try to take advantage of it. Your first urge should be an urge to protect what has been given to you to guard, because it is valuable to me and it is mine. Period."

What we ask of slaves is not easy: Be entirely open to Me, and yet have good boundaries with the rest of the world. Many have trouble with the switching back and forth; they want to be one or the other, and they overcompensate in one area, or mess up. They need help and practice in getting this right.

Q: My sub doesn't know when to keep her mouth shut. When strangers online ask her personal questions that I'd rather not have answered, she just tells them. I expected her to use some discretion!

Raven: Once you've actually communicated with her enough to understand why she feels like she has to be obedient to strangers, and figured out a way to get her to understand (and agree) that she should be submissive only to you (if that's what you want), then you may need to be more specific about what "discretion" means.

My boy and I had to work this one out together. In establishing the idea of "discretion", we had to decide what of whose personal information is not ill-advised to disclose to whom. Friends, and how close, and in what demographic? Family? People at his school? People at his job? Strangers on a website? Do they get to know about my/his/our: Sexual preferences? Gender status? Religion? Sexual proclivities? M/s lifestyle? Age? Political opinions? Profession? Marital status? Size of genitalia? Existence of children? Home address? Phone number? Medical status?

We went over every item that might create problems for disclosure, and each place where it should or should not be disclosed, and what he should do if he discovered that someone now knew about something unexpectedly, or if he really wanted to disclose something to someone. As the owner, making clear guidelines for your property as to what is and is not acceptable helps them do their job better, and keeps you from getting shot in the foot through lack of planning ahead. (Whenever you encounter areas where there are differing assumptions between master and slave, I strongly encourage putting these details in writing for the sub to refer to when necessary.)

Sometimes, instead of looking for something to blame and punish in the s-type, the D-type needs to say to themselves, "I'm the one in charge. The buck stops here. Was there something that I didn't do that contributed to this problem? Where am *I* responsible?" Then go do something about it.

Q: Should the goal of a slave be to have no desires of their own? Doesn't that seem kind of impossible? And what if I like it that my slave has some individual desires of their own?

Raven: Do I think that the end-goal for them is to learn to let go of their own desires and align themselves entirely with the owner? Yes, that's kind of the point. Not easy? Damn straight it isn't easy, regardless of whether you are doing it for your owner or for oneness with the Universe. But then who said that any worthwhile calling was ever easy? (And yes, I would use the word *calling* for a strong, clean, core drive for service and/or submission.)

However, as with all worthwhile callings, it is a work in progress. I think that the correct way to put it is not that "slaves should not have desires", but that slaves should be *continually working towards* letting go of desires that conflict with them doing their path with a whole heart, and also towards aligning their desires with those of their owners. This isn't going to happen overnight, or even in a decade. It's a long slow process. A slave can't be ordered to lose their desires by tomorrow or next week, any more than they can be ordered to lose 50 pounds by next week. It's not going to happen without a lot of striving, and of course the light bulb has to really want to change.

The first thing that they have to internalize is the owner's priorities as to which of their desires need to be altered now, which can wait until later in the process, and which are irrelevant and can remain ... but even those last ones remain by leave of the owner, and as such become part of the owner's "plan" for the slave. For example, I knew nothing of yoga before I met Joshua, but after seeing how much it helps him, I have now made it part of his regular plan. It probably would have been anyway, but I've "approved" it now.

Joshua came to me with X array of desires, seven years ago. His desire for hot perverted sex, for example, or alphabetizing the pantry, not only need not be changed, but can be put squarely in the service of the enslavement. His desire for avocadoes (he bought some last night as a treat for himself) is utterly irrelevant to his enslavement and I see no reason to do anything with it. His desire for Sudoku or computer games is irrelevant only so long as it does not interfere with what I want him to do, so rather than change those desires, I simply implement other programming that says, "These must be put aside if I am called. They are less important than my master's needs." His desire for rampant promiscuous (and rather unsafe) sex with all manner of strangers, on the other hand, had to go. Those are just some examples of the "sorting mechanism" that had to happen with everything he did or wanted. Not that I'm done with it. Not at all. It is still very much a work in progress.

The Bonsai Tree:
Shaping A Slave

Discipline

Q: How would you punish your slave for disobedience?

Raven: We are very unusual in the D/s and M/s demographic in that we don't use a punishment context at all. Before I go on to describe what we do instead, I should say that we are aware that the majority of D/s and M/s folks do use punishment, and that we've talked to an awful lot of them about it in order to answer this question ... which does come up pretty often.

If I caught my slave deliberately doing something that I had forbidden him to do, the punishment would be a long, arduous processing session during which we would discuss whether or not this relationship and this power dynamic was working after all, or whether we should call the whole thing off. Frankly, if he does not obey my commands, then his obedience to me doesn't mean all that much, does it? And in that case, I don't want to be doing this with him, and maybe he should run along and find a master who will just do fetishy stuff with him and not expect real commitment to service.

As far as I am concerned, if we are in a real M/s relationship, then he will want to obey me completely—which he does—with every part of his heart. The worst punishment I've ever used was sending him away to sleep elsewhere, cutting off contact for a day. That has always worked. Usually the only punishment I ever need to give him is to express how incredibly disappointed I am in him. If the M/s bond is real, that should be all that is necessary to reduce a slave to abject misery.

I consider it a privilege to serve me—I'm an honorable and ethical master, and working for me means supporting all sorts of greater goals in the world—so if a slave is being continually rebellious, I might assume that they are no longer interested in that privilege. Generally, though, if an order isn't carried out, something else is probably wrong. Perhaps they forgot, or overextended themselves, or had other troubles. It's my job to help them figure out what went wrong, and figure out how it can be fixed, and help them with that process.

However, there are slaves out there who really love and require the punishment system. After having talked to a lot of them, I've found that they tended to have the following reasons:

1) Some slaves really like to rebel and be slapped down because it reminds them of who's in charge. I am thankful that there are owners who are willing to take on these rebellious types.

2) I've also heard from slaves who found physical punishment to be useful in that it gave them a way to expiate their guilt at failing their owners, even in small ways. For them, the punishment gave them some peace of mind, expiating their bad feelings on the matter and giving them a physical catharsis. I can see how it could be useful as atonement for such people, as long as the owner did it in a clean way. (That wouldn't work for me, because making my slave suffer—while potentially very hot—does not actually alleviate my anger and disappointment in regard to their error. The only thing that works for that is seeing them refrain from doing the wrong thing for a period of time.)

3) Some slaves act out when they are having a bad time emotionally, and they really want a catharsis. The physical punishment gives them what they need. While my own personal preference might be to train a slave to be mindful when this need arose and ask for a catharsis before anything went awry, many owners don't seem to mind this situation, and simply allow the slave to remain unconscious of why they are acting out, and give them their beating without making a psychological production of it. My worry in this situation would be that this can condition the slave into a pattern of "I feel crappy for other reasons, I know that a catharsis will help, I act out, I get one, next time feeling crappy will trigger me to act out again." This is more subtle and unconscious than "I like spankings and maybe if I act out Mistress will spank me as a fake "punishment". The punishment is honestly unpleasant to

the slave, as is pissing off their M-type, but they feel good enough afterwards that they will come to crave it. This makes the owner into the pusher from whom they get their "fix".

Joshua: My master made it clear from the beginning that the only punishment for willful disobedience is his grave disappointment, and being sat down for a long conversation about what went wrong. For the second offense, I would be sent away from him for a time, isolated from the privilege of serving him. I have rarely been willfully disobedient, so I suppose you could say it is an effective deterrent. I know exactly what I can expect from him, and what he expects from me, and I like that.

I've only screwed up a few times so badly that I was dragged out for a formal lecture. Usually if I make mistakes it is through incompetence or inattention, and he just treats me like defective machinery and figures out how these mistakes can be avoided in the future. Two or three times he's gotten so irritated with me that he sent me away and had me sleep in the treehouse. (That part of it wasn't punishment, because I like sleeping in the treehouse.) It was the knowledge that he didn't want me around right then that was the real punishment.

Q: Is it OK if I get turned on by punishing my slave and watching him suffer, or should punishment always be nonsexual and not about gratification for me?

Raven: That's a hard question, and one that I've seen bitterly fought over. There are those who say that the dominant's attitude during punishment ought be somber and serious, and that enjoying making the sub suffer should only be done separately for play.

Others say that they get turned on during punishments, and enjoy it, and there's nothing wrong with it. I think that it can work if both parties are very self-aware and mindful, but except for those few cases I worry about possible conditioning.

It's not just the dominant who might be subtly encouraged to look a little harder and a little more irrationally for faults in order to get some pleasure out of it. I worry about the reactions of a sub who desperately wants to please their dominant being in a situation where even a hated punishment after a bad infraction becomes associated with the dominant's visible pleasure. I'd say: Approach with care, and make sure you understand what messages are being given to your sub, and to your subconscious.

A (very) few of the dominants I know have chosen as slave-punishment activities that also inconvenience (or in some cases actively hurt) them as well. The dominant is choosing to be pained by the punishment, and endures it as a matter of honor. In these cases the punishment is not only unambiguously negative, but it adds a clear picture of the dominant's suffering on top of the other pain or deprivation. This only works with dominants who are very self-disciplined and submissives who are deeply moved by such things, however.

Q: My Mistress keeps punishing me for all sorts of things. It seems like she'll punish me at the drop of a hat! I left the margarine out, and got punished, and was told that I ought to know better. I don't understand, and I'm afraid that I am just going to keep screwing up all the time.

Raven: First of all, has your mistress been clear with you as to what the rules are? Is she willing to put them down in writing for you? There's no point in punishing you for rules that have not been made clear … right down to how to treat margarine. If your responsibility is to follow the rules, at least one of her complementary responsibilities is listing them in a way that is concise and easily available to you while you are learning them. If she can't be bothered to do that, then she will have to put up with a lot more mistakes.

Second, have you discussed with your mistress what the purposes of her punishments are? What is her theory of behavior modification? Has she tried it on anyone before? What were the results? If she's a new dominant, you're going to end up in the position of "guinea pig" and she's bound to make some mistakes. If she's an honorable person, she will hopefully be able to acknowledge them and change. It might be good if the two of you sat down and discussed what she actually hopes to accomplish with the punishments, and whether this is the sort of thing that is likely to work on you. Different slaves require different approaches; there's no one big perfect slave training manual that applies to all of them.

For example, if she is trying to use corporal punishment as a means to modify your behavior, she has to be consistent about that. It can't be done just because either of you thinks it's fun, or emotionally satisfying. She can't be looking for a fault in you just to have an excuse to whale on you. If there's any of that in her motivation, she'll drive you crazy, and not in a good way. That's a fun game for part-time play D/s—"Oh, you've been bad, you couldn't balance six golf clubs on your head while bringing me a drink, I'd better break out the cane and punish you now." But it has no place in real life.

This is something that I have trouble getting across to people who graduate, as it were, from play D/s to real D/s—a slaveowner doesn't need an excuse to whale on the slave. They can—and should—do it openly as "Because I want to; because it pleases me to do it; this isn't about you or your behavior, it's about my pleasure." It's even healthier to do it as "I'm in a really bad mood and I want to hit something, and you're the only one that I can hit," than to deliberately find fault with the slave. The problem is that for some dominants, there is great pleasure not just in the sadism of beating someone, but in the satisfaction of the righteousness that one feels in "justly punishing" someone, and punishment can sometimes be more about them seeking that satisfaction than actually trying to change the submissive. If they really want to play mind-games, well, we address that later in this section.

If, however, she really is trying to use it only as behavior modification—and you guys need to talk about whether using it as behavior modification is going to mess with doing it for fun—then she should follow this up by finding out if it really worked or not. What do you think that she meant for you to learn by this? Is that what you absorbed? How will it change your behavior in the future? Do either of you think that it will make you do things differently? Is that what she was trying to instill, or was she going for a bigger lesson that had nothing to do with margarine? If so, did you get it? If you didn't, she needs to know that. For that matter, is your mistress absolutely set on physical-pain punishments? Does she have any reason for that other than this is what all the slaveowners in porn stories do? Has she talked to other owners about different types of behavior modification, and how to figure out what's right for what slave?

There's another point in there too. While she technically has the right to punish you for something as trivial as leaving out the margarine, does she have a realistic view of how perfect (as in never, ever making any mistakes) it is possible for you to get? You're still human. You will never become so perfect that you never screw up anything. You're not a robot. Have you discussed with her the standards as to what mistakes are too trivial to warrant more than a reprimand, or is she enthusiastic about beating you daily for every tiny flaw?

I realize that these are all things that are really up to her to consider, but perhaps you should suggest talking about them? It seems like there are some communication breakdowns with regard to expectations, standards, and long-term goals for your training. If she doesn't keep you posted, it will be much more difficult for you to help her to change you properly.

Q: When the slave is having a hard time, should the master back off on them, or push them?

Raven: That's a tough one, and one of the most delicate and difficult decisions that a slaveowner can make ... and you are guaranteed to make mistakes in that arena. That's all right; mistakes are human. But it has to be judged on a slave-by-slave, and sometimes a case-by-case, basis. If a slave is in a really bad way for some reason, and you decide to push them, and they try hard and fail anyway, you as the owner need to take half the credit for that failure. You'll also need to make it clear to them that you don't hold it against them.

On the other side, if you spare them the duty, that can be a wonderful act of mercy ... or not. It depends on the slave in question. Some slaves have unrealistic expectations of themselves, and those are the ones who will chafe when you say, "No, you can't finish that tonight. You're exhausted. Go to bed." They'll chafe even if you're right, even if they'd make themselves ill by finishing the task, or even if you can see that it's not possible. For those slaves it's especially important that you make it clear to them that you, not they, are the one whose judgment will be counted regarding their ability to do anything.

Joshua: From experience, I'll tell you that backing off often isn't really the greater mercy. In the beginning, my master frequently backed off when I was struggling with something. He'd just lower his expectations. At first, this was a great relief, but over time I felt more and more incompetent, like I obviously couldn't be expected to come through on anything. Eventually it got to a point where I got angry at him for expecting so little of me. (He's said that he knew I would respond well to the challenge of "I'll show you!") Then he started building the expectations up again, and I was both relieved and scared. It was a really difficult pattern for me to work through, but now when I really wish he'd back off on an order, I can remember where that road leads, and I'm grateful for his strictness. But I think I really needed to walk that road in order to get to the point of gratitude without resentment.

Q: Should you punish a slave for forgetfulness? Will it help them to remember?

Raven: I was punished frequently as a child for forgetting to do things, and it never seemed fair to me, as there had never been any deliberate disobedience on my part, and punishing me for forgetting never seemed to do a damn bit of good as far as I could tell when it came to making me remember things better. If anything, being nervous and jittery and worried about punishment made me more likely to screw up and forget things. So I treat forgetfulness differently. (For tips on dealing with a slave who has neurological or chemical disorders, see the section on Obstacles.)

I think that some masters have an idea that if they punish a slave for forgetting X, then X will have a charged memory attached to it, and they won't forget X again (although nothing says that they won't forget Y, and I personally think that you can only do that so many times). Maybe it works for some folks, maybe not for others.

If the problem is that the slave is continually forgetting one particular thing, then some deep work needs to be done in their psyche to figure out what's going on. Often, when probing, I find that what's really happening is that they secretly believe that what they're being asked to do is stupid, or not the "right" way to go about it (meaning what they think ought to be done) and that vague contempt for their owner's "bad" decision leaks upward from the subconscious and causes them to forget to do whatever it was. That's passive-aggressive, and should be rooted out and stopped.

One can also work on associating the easily-forgotten thing with something else. "Every time you look at X, you're going to remember Y." This requires the owner to keep reminding them about it until it sticks.

Q: My master wants me to beg for things, and I do try, but he says that it doesn't sound sincere! No matter how hard I try, he says it's not good enough and then punishes me! What should I do? Take acting lessons? I've asked him to help, but he just grins and tells me to try harder. I haven't had an orgasm in two weeks because I haven't been able to beg well enough to "earn" one!

Raven: Frankly, it sounds like your master is messing with you for his own entertainment. If he really knows you well, he will be able to figure out quickly when you're sincere or not. If he doesn't know you well enough to know that, then he shouldn't be judging your level of sincerity until he does. But from what you've said—the refusal to help you, liking to watch you struggle with it—this sounds like he's deliberately setting you up for failure for his own sadistic entertainment.

Now, lest you think I'm saying "evil naughty master" ... I'm not. If you agreed to be his submissive, then he has the right to entertain himself at your expense. (Unless you two have negotiated things otherwise.) Emotional sadism, tormenting the submissive with games they can't win for the owner's amusement ... this is par for the course for many D/s relationships, especially the sexual parts. If this is the case, then the lesson here is not that you need to learn to beg more realistically ... it's that you need to:

❖ Learn that your orgasms, in these cases, are not your own, and can be denied at your owner's whim. Learn to be OK with that, in the end. It may be that he hasn't yet gotten around to understanding that he can deny your orgasms for any reason, including "I think it's funny", and has to make up fake excuses—"you weren't begging well enough"—to pretend to justify it. Or, perhaps, he knows that perfectly well and it's just more entertaining with fake excuses. Either way, you need to let go of the idea that there is any sure way to "earn" or "win" orgasms. There isn't. They aren't yours, and you can't "win" against your master anyway. If he decides to be merciful and grant you one, consider yourself lucky. If he doesn't, that's just the way things are. No, it isn't fair. Fair isn't the *point* here. Control, and giving up that control with inner grace, is the point.

❖ Learn to see entertaining your master with your anguished struggles as a service to him. You'd prance around in scanty longerie for him, right? You'd do a sexy strip-dance if he ordered it, right? You'd rent his favorite movie and watch it with him, even if you hate it, right? (If you wouldn't do these things for him, maybe you need to rethink your chosen position in this relationship?) Being visibly frustrated is just part of that entertainment. It's just another service. Instead of offering him your body or your works to be amused by, you're offering him your emotions.

❖ If possible, learn to eroticize being actively sexually frustrated by him. If you can learn to love it as least as much as you hate it, you'll manage better.

❖ Learn to discern when something is just frustrating you (but you can handle it) and when something is really screwing with you, and learn how you can respectfully bring the latter to him—perhaps "Sir, that thing X that you do is really making me feel bad about myself, and I want to cry and I feel depressed whenever I think about it. Could you help me understand why it's necessary, and help me through the hard parts?"

I know that for particularly service-oriented slaves, being set up for failure, even if they know it's for the owner's entertainment, is very rough on their self-esteem and they need a lot of help to get through that. (I also know that it's difficult for control-oriented slaves who are having a hard time giving up control, difficult for entirely different reasons.) I have a very service-oriented boy, and I make sure never to play this game outside of our sex life. During sex, though, anything goes, and it's all about entertaining me, even if it means emotional sadism. The boundary comforts him, lets him know where he stands in daily life, and helps him not to take sexual teasing personally. I have done things like sexually tease him for a hour, and then say, "Never mind. Go to sleep," and rolled over, jerked off, and gone to sleep myself. He now knows that his obvious discomfort and frustration pleases me, and he's learned to eroticize that. But if he told me that it was really fucking with his head in a bad way, and he meant it, I would rethink things.

I realize that emotional sadism as entertainment can be a rough thing for a new slave to fully understand, and to reconcile with an otherwise caring master. But it might behoove you to observe him closely, and watch how he does things, watch his motivations. After all, if one has that urge, where can one put it except for a willing slave? It's a great service to offer: "You can mess with me and make me squirm and cry, and I'm sturdy enough not to be damaged by it, and submissive enough to enjoy the control, and self-aware enough to know that it's just a game, and I won't tell you that you suck for wanting it."

However, as we've mentioned in previous questions, this kind of thing can be crazy-making for the slave if it's not openly discussed. At the very least, the dominant should make clear boundaries around it—"During the day, when I want you to do something, I expect excellence in the task. If I take out the whip and start a scene at night, however, I expect you to do your best and be a good sport about whatever happens, and your measure of excellence should be based on how much I'm enjoying myself rather than how well you did on any given task."

Joshua: I've been on the receiving end of this sort of thing with various dominants over the years. For some, it's clearly just a game, and they aren't trying to convince you that it's all that important. Other dominants want it to be taken much more seriously, because it creates a more satisfying reaction.

However, a small minority of the latter group do cross the line into abuse. How to tell the abusive ones? From what I've seen, they tend to deliberately pick submissives who don't have the emotional resources to deal with it. They don't limit it to bedroom activities; it pervades every aspect of the slave's life. They won't talk about it honestly, either, but always pretend that it's perfectly reasonable. On the other hand, when it is clearly just a game for the dominant and they're honest about that, the dominants often actually enjoy when the submissives figure it out. It doesn't stop the game, because they're banking on you going along with it anyway.

Assuming that you have a dominant who isn't being abusive with it, but who sees it as entertainment, learning how to play this game with grace involves developing detachment about the outcome. You can't be invested in your success or failure. It can become a powerful opportunity for self-growth— you do your best, keep a good attitude, know that the outcome is out of your control, and do it anyway. It's very Zen-like in its own way. Of course, there's always the danger that if you manage to pull off that kind of serene equanimity, some dominants may lose interest, because the struggle is what they're looking for.

Q: My slave says that he wants more rules and protocol, but I think it's stupid and a waste of my time. It seems like a lot of work for me—coming up with rules, constantly enforcing them, and for what? I don't get anything out of it. Can't we just have a M/s relationship without rules and protocol?

Raven: I know how you feel, because I felt that way myself in the beginning. My boy is the sort who loves rules and protocol, the more the better. He'd be happy living like a monk with every day carefully planned out and exactly the same. I'm not like that. I thrive on variety, and my jobs and life reflect that. He's had to make some adjustments ... but so have I. If a slave is expected to live by the owner's rules, it's not fair to them not to have those rules written down where they can refer to them. And as for protocols ... well, a protocol is simply an "If X, then do Y." It's useful to have those around, especially when the owner isn't present to ask.

The problem comes in when the owner, the slave, and the BDSM culture have different ideas about what sorts of protocol are the "right" way to do things. When I went looking for rules and protocols, I found a lot of them ... and none of them did anything for me. When Joshua begged me for protocols, I tried various ones out, and I found quickly that if it didn't feel like it was doing something really useful for me—something that I'd seriously miss if it went away—I couldn't bring myself to regularly and consistently enforce them, and they would fall by the wayside.

The first step, for me, was that I had to get to the point of not feeling that I was a bad dominant if I had no use for all the sorts of protocols that all the other dominants seemed to be using. Then I had to get *him* to the point of not feeling that I was a bad dominant if I had no use for the sort of protocols that all the other dominants seemed to be using. That took a little longer. (It is probably becoming obvious to the reader that the "traditional" aesthetic rules of D/s play were the opposite of helpful for us in working out the structure of our dynamic.)

For a time we had very few rules and protocols, except for a few large overarching ones. This made Joshua unhappy, but it also created confusion when he wasn't sure what action applied to what situation. So for two years, I worked quietly on the problem. Whenever any ordinary situation went wrong, or created conflict, or annoyed me, I would ask myself, "Is there something that Joshua could have done to prevent this or change the outcome?" This included situations that weren't specifically to do with him, such as the car nearly running out of gas. Then, finally, I created a list of rules and protocols that used Joshua as a tool to improve these situations. It improved them to the point where I was motivated to correct their absence. This was something I could get behind, a system that made less work for me rather than more work, even taking into account the time and effort spent correcting his errors. For someone who thought of himself as low-protocol, it's amazing how many pages of rules I came up with.

It's something that is almost never taught to beginning dominants: how do you create your own rules based on your life's needs and not on anyone else's system? It's a long process, because most of us are raised to be fairly self-sufficient, and in our pre-mastery lives we often got used to doing it ourselves or doing without. There are very few resources to help us figure out how to create slave systems that make our lives easier, instead of merely making our slaves feel slavier. If I'd had that sort of mentoring, it would have spared us a lot of trouble in the beginning.

Q: How do you get a slave to remember their rules and protocols? My girl keeps forgetting to do them. Should I cut back and not have so many? How many is too many to remember?

Raven: That depends on the slave in question, of course. However, it also depends on how fast and how thoroughly you want them to learn your rules. I don't mind taking a long time with the process, while some owners prefer a steeper learning curve, perhaps to weed out the unsuitable. My goal with regard to rules is to have Joshua eventually internalize every rule. It should go from "I do this because this is the way my master wants it done" to "I do this because it's the right way for me to do it; was there ever any other way?" What I've found to be most useful is to take a selection of the rules—perhaps the ones that are currently most relevant, about 20 of them—and concentrate on those. I have him set up a chart of eight weeks with those rules, and he marks an X where he's messed up. This gives him a clear picture of where he needs work, and helps both of us realistically track his progress.

There is no punishment for the demerit—it's an assessment tool—but if he racks up a number of demerits under any one rule, we sit down and figure out why this one is so hard for him, and how it could be made easier. When the X's taper off and he has a clean eight-week period with a rule, we put it aside and install another one. If it starts to go wrong again, it gets an assessment and goes back up.

Some owners do prefer to use a punishment context, for reasons discussed under that question. But no matter what motivation is used, having a clear and open way for both dominant and submissive to keep track of progress is important. So is patience. Remember that it's all right for this to take years. Internalizing of rules on a deep level takes years anyway. How to tell if a rule is internalized? Send them away for a week and see which rules they continue to follow, or feel extremely uncomfortable that they are not able to follow. If they quickly forget it, it's not internalized.

Transparency

Q: Is it really necessary for the owner to know everything about the slave? What if they're made uncomfortable by that much invasiveness?

Raven: Yes, it is that necessary. And that's as it should be...not just for romantic reasons. It should be that way because *this is the way to make it work*. Without knowing the slave that deeply, the owner cannot hope to fully enslave them. You can't drive a car blindfolded, or with the windshield covered. You can drive it with the instrument panel covered, for a while anyway, but stuff will start fairly quickly to go wrong out of "nowhere". While you can drive it for a good while without ever knowing anything about the mechanism under the hood, when it does inevitably go wrong, you've got to hire a professional to fix it for you, and that's just not a option for most people who are attempting M/s. (Certainly when I've been that professional, one of the first things I'll do is to call the couple on that. "Why the heck *aren't* you telling them this? And why aren't *you* giving them no peace until you get that out of them?") We call this transparency, meaning that the slave must be entirely transparent to the owner, and we don't do it for fun and romance. We do it because it's necessary to achieve what we want.

I would think that if a would-be slave is feeling ill at ease with the transparency, they are not comfortable with being owned to that extent, and that needs to be talked about. If the slave is just having some problems adjusting, well, *not* being transparent about that, and negotiating things out will just make it worse until it blows up.

I've often said that while there are various rules in our contract that I could live without (wouldn't like it, but I could deal) the real dealbreaker is the following one:

Part II: Absolute access to Mind. Joshua has no right to privacy of word, thought, or deed from his master. Raven can demand and expect to get immediate and truthful information on any part of Joshua's life, including dreams, thoughts, fantasies, information, knowledge, and words and deeds past and present. Anything that Joshua knows, thinks, or writes will be at Raven's disposal.

We put this contract together before either of us ever heard of the terms TPE, or IE, or transparency. All I knew was that in order to make this thing work for him as well as me, I had to have access to as much of his thoughts and feelings as I possibly could, period. Without this, there is no way that it would feel like actual mastery. It would feel like limited D/s ... which isn't a bad thing, but isn't what we decided that we wanted.

It wasn't easy at first. Joshua is a reserved, cynical, untrusting person with a whole lot of barriers. He had spent most of his life ignoring his feelings except when it was impossible to do so, and had few skills in analyzing them. I had to do a lot of remedial emotional training in the beginning, teaching him to notice and report his feelings before they built up in his subconscious and began to sabotage his actions. And yes, that meant a *lot* of questions I had to ask, a lot of interrogation. Fortunately I'm the sort who likes to know how people tick, so it was interesting to me, not just a chore.

Sometimes I had him do writing assignments on various things related his inner workings. Sometimes I just told him to think about a thing for a few days and get back to me on it by a certain time. Perhaps it might have gone easier if I had been working with someone who had more emotional skills and experience, but then again I've had much worse—Joshua was far less damaged and traumatized than many of my former lovers; it was about learning, not years of unlearning.

I do find it ironic that much so-called "slave training" seems to be designed to make "slaves" less mindful of themselves and their motivations, rather than more so. I really think that "enslaving" systems that encourage the slaves to ignore their own feelings are doomed. Attitude is very important to being a good slave, but it can't be surface attitude; it has to be honestly felt all the way down. To put that in place requires a good deal of self-knowledge—you can't collude in changing yourself (and all slave training should be a collusion between M and s) if you don't know what's there and how best to move it around. In fact, one of the best gifts that a submissive can give a new dominant is a great deal of previous introspection and self-knowledge—having the manual already written, as it were.

But most people aren't trained to be able to handle transparency. In theory, it sounds good, but in practice, they freeze up. (What, you mean you really want to know all of me, even the stuff that I know you'll find icky? But how can I know that you won't reject me for that?) And, in truth, what if they do reveal something to you that you don't like? What's the most effective reaction? By effective, I mean the reaction that's going to get them to want to reveal other difficult things, not the one that will merely encourage more desperate cover-ups. It's something to think about. The owner needs to be willing to accept the awful things that might be said without reacting personally. One of the best gifts a dominant can give a submissive (to turn the issue around) is the assurance that even the worst parts of them will be accepted with equanimity and not with revulsion.

Anyway, the first period of our relationship allowed him to say anything to me, in any tone of voice, with any wording, so long as it was in private. (Well, I did forbid him to swear at me, largely because it was amusing to watch him struggle with that.) But this was important, because it got him into the habit of really understanding that anything he thinks or feels is my property. It's all mine, and it is his duty to offer it all to me. His lifelong habits of emotional repression and reserve and isolation took quite a while to overcome, as well as getting rid of the idea that I wouldn't really want to know about *those* thoughts, they were terrible and unflattering and he ought to keep them to himself. No. I don't care how awful the thought is, I want to know about it, and it is mine by right of our agreement. It's not for him to decide which thoughts I do or don't want to know about. Even if it's "Raven sucks, and all I really want to do today is yell at him and tell him how much he sucks." That too.

Also, I feel that it was important during this time to build up his trust in my ability to gracefully handle being told about these sorts of things. Being able to say, "Honestly, right now all I can think about is all the things you do that tick me off, like X and Y and Z..." and have the owner respond calmly and not angrily, that's crucial. No matter how dominant you are, you can't order deep trust to appear. You have to earn it, and then continue to keep it.

Then we started putting in rules about how these things could be said, and how often they could be brought up, and under what circumstances. Now that he's had years to get used to telling me everything, and having that feel natural, we can carefully channel that flow of information to be more respectful, without censoring the content. This is because being rude to me is bad for him emotionally; it makes him feel worse about himself, and the external wall of a rule of respect helps him feel more in control.

Frankly, I have my own anger management issues, but I'm a public figure in charge of a lot of people, and I can't afford to get peeved because someone I'm in charge of speaks to me disrespectfully. I don't own them, or their mouths. So I decided to use that period of time when he could (and did) freely say awful things to me as a way to hone my own internal discipline. I mean, if you can't hear that stuff from your slave, who is in a position of extreme vulnerability to you, what does that say about the fragility of your ego? So even there I used him, and his struggle, as a sort of spiritual "sparring partner" to work on my own issue, because I hate to waste anything. It was useful and valuable for both of us, in terms of mindfulness for me and openness for him, but now we have moved on. I can trust him to not use courtesy and submission as a way to hide from me, and he trusts me to be able to maturely hear uncomfortable things, and now he can have communication rules without censoring himself.

If the slave gets to a point where they can appreciate the honesty, it makes things easier, because you can say, "So I know that you love it when I'm honest, and you'd hate knowing that I was holding back something because I was afraid of your reaction. So I'm going to say something to you now that is probably going to hurt, the sort of thing that the sensitive types would probably get all bent out of shape over and wish I'd lied about. But you're not like that, so I can give you the privilege of the full extent of my thoughts, even ones I wouldn't say to other people. You can be that for me in a way that they can't."

Cuts down on possible slave drama, let me tell you. Only had to say it twice, in the beginning. And yes, I meant every word of it.

Joshua: I don't think I could be enslaved without transparency. Like Raven said, I am a guarded, paranoid person. I am intensely private about my inner stuff; the public "me" is very different than the inner me. People often think they know me better than they really do, or think I am being more emotionally vulnerable than I really am. Because I do public speaking about sex, gender, BDSM, spirituality, and so forth, I have "declassified" huge sections of what for most people is very intimate, private information. That's no longer intimate for me. My private stuff is elsewhere.

Someone who wants to get inside my head needs to understand that, and be able to see through it. They need to be able to look at my carefully polished "intimate" disclosure and say, "Yeah, that's part of it. Where's the rest?" To be owned, I need my master to have that kind of access. I can easily render obedient service without deep internal submission. I don't need to be controlled to obey; I'm obedient by nature ... but inside I am untouched. If he would allow it, it would be a point of honor for me to show my master nothing of my internal struggle. That's perfect service, but not slavery. To have no privacy—not even in the darkest corners of my own self—is what being owned is about for me. Power I'll give up readily, but my emotional privacy I guard. Giving that up was a painful process for me, and I had to start small.

My master expects complete radical honesty from me and absolutely no right to privacy. Anything I think he'd be interested in knowing, or that I'd rather him not know, I'm obligated to tell him. In fact, one of his favorite terrifying questions is "What have you been thinking about lately that you'd rather I not know about?" I can say what I like to others, but I have to be mindful that my behavior reflects on him.

He's promised to be entirely honest with me in all matters, and that if he wants privacy regarding a certain issue, he'll say that plainly. I really like this. It makes it so much easier for me to have an emotionally intimate relationship with him. I'm naturally paranoid about these things, so if I know that he'll tell me what is really going on, no matter how unpleasant, then I don't have to fret about what terrible things he *might* be thinking. Besides, I can usually tell that there is something going on, and my paranoid speculation is almost always far worse than what it really is. (Many times someone has made a big "confession" to me and I've had to restrain my impulse to say "Is that all? Why'd you get so worked up about that?") With my master, I'm absolutely not expected to coddle his ego regarding anything, although I am also not supposed to be thoughtlessly critical or say intentionally hurtful things. I try to give a fair assessment. But then again, he doesn't ever ask people questions that he doesn't want honest answers to.

Is it worth it? Well, the radical honesty *is* the payoff, really. It means that I have no reason to hide anything from him. He accepts and loves me, knowing all the creepy hard-to-love stuff about me. I don't have to hide a single thing, fearing that he'll reject me. I don't have to worry about presenting myself to him in the most appealing way. Or rather, when I present myself to him in an appealing way, I know that he can see through it. He might appreciate the presentation, but he doesn't mistake it for the whole.

Being praised and valued for something that is only a small piece of who you are becomes hollow over time. It reaffirms the nagging suspicion that who you really are isn't as valuable as your mask. With my master, I can be entirely genuine. He can see me as I really am, which means that I can better see myself, and that's entirely worth it. After having experienced this, I would never choose to have privacy from him, even if he offered it.

On the other hand, I don't know if I could have done radical honesty without D/s. Not only would I refuse to offer this freely, I couldn't have done it with someone whom I was *able* to deceive. Frankly, I do not have the strictest ethics. My desire for privacy overrides any sense of obligation I feel to be strictly honest when it comes to deeply personal things. I needed someone I could not deceive even when I tried, and I may be a sneaky little weasel, but I am no match for my master. Frankly, concealing myself and being called out for it is so much more humiliating than just laying it out there. It's interesting to look back on it and realize that even though we both knew he could, he never directly pushed me to reveal myself . He is subtle. Instead of ripping my off metaphorical clothing or ordering me to strip, he just commented, "You're still wearing X." And he waited.

Giving my master access to my journal was a big step for me, early on. I could easily show him deeply intimate (even for me) writing that I did when I knew ahead of time he would read it, but it was different for him to read things I'd written under the assumption that no one would never see them. At first, he only asked if I would mind showing it to him. I balked, told him I'd really rather not. He accepted that and didn't press me, but told me to think about whether I could trust him with it. Months later I gave it to him, because I realized that it was his by right, and it was wrong for me to want to hold it back from him. If he had taken it from me, I think I would have resented it, and it would have felt like a violation. It isn't that I object so terribly to being violated, but violation implies resistance, a lack of right to whatever it is you are taking. Violation is a fun sex game, but in "real life" he expects me to yield without hesitation. Early on I hesitated a good deal, but I always yielded. Now I don't even think about it. I still have my big emotional walls and things I'd rather not discuss with anyone, but my master doesn't count as "anyone".

Q: On the other side ... I worry about the slave knowing too much about the owner. What happens when the slave can second-guess the owner so well that they just do everything they want without being asked? Could that be considered topping from the bottom in some way?

Raven: Assuming that you've done this right, and this person is now spending huge amounts of attention trying to figure out what it is that you like, in order to please you ... then how is this topping from the bottom? A smart submissive will quickly realize "My owner doesn't like it when I top from the bottom, and these actions come across that way. So I won't do that." An experienced slave will figure out: "My owner doesn't want me to top from the bottom, and really I don't want that either, partly because I want what they want, and partly because I know that this M/s relationship won't work if I try that. So I won't. My priorities are making this go the way the owner wants."

I can't imagine how that could be challenging someone's authority. Of course, an insecure and paranoid owner might worry that if the slave knew them really well they'd try to manipulate them, but that's the owner not having faith in their own ability to train the slave out of that. And maybe that's true! If you're realistically realizing that you are an inexperienced owner with an intelligent and manipulative slave, and you've completely lost control of the situation because they know you well enough to push your buttons and make you "enslave" them in the way that they want, with no real inconvenience to them, well, maybe it needs to end, or you need to figure out a way to take back control and keep it.

Joshua: I'd add that if the slave seems at all inclined to this type of manipulation, they might benefit from a period of time where they had little (if any) input into how things would be done, and they were not permitted to act except under direct orders.

Doormats and Misbehaving Slaves

Q: Should a slave be a total doormat? Is this what masters want? Or do they want a certain amount of disobedience? What if they want a feisty slave? Or even a bratty one?

Raven: By definition, the perfect slave (if there were such a beast) would do whatever their owner wanted. If their owner wanted them to resist a certain percentage of orders (for entertainment, perhaps? for an excuse to "punish" them?) or question certain orders (because the owner wants the slave's perspective on things), then the owner would let the slave know, overtly or covertly, and the perfect slave would do it ... therefore tacitly doing whatever the owner wants, still.

I've occasionally known an owner to want a slave who was continually outright disobedient. I've known a few who wanted slaves to pretend rebellion for the fun of being wrestled down, as it were. One owner openly told me that a slave who never disobeyed in order to provoke punishment would not be interesting to him; he really enjoyed the challenge of asserting his dominance over and over with a "difficult" slave. This was an eye-opening perspective for me, as I'm personally very far to the side of "perfect slave means absolute obedience". So a submissive who is highly invested in an independent persona might want to actively seek out a dominant who enjoys the thrill of the takedown more than the "boring" comfort of dependable obedience.

As to the problem of outright brattiness (which term Joshua once defined as being "charmingly disobedient"), I have no problem with subs who are continually bratty ... as long as they belong to someone else who wants that sort of thing, and I don't have to be in charge of them. For me, allowing my slave to help me with the important things in my life requires placing a lot of trust in them, and I don't trust easily. I prefer a slave that I can solidly depend on without worrying if they're going to rebel at the worst possible moment and ruin things for me. I also depend on a slave for positive companionship and safe intimacy, and for me personally, brattiness would make me less likely to want to be open with them. Continually disobeying or being disrespectful would have me saying soberly that it is clear that we aren't right for each other, we're not a good fit together, and I will release you to find someone better suited for that sort of thing. I think that fit and suitability is the basis of M/s—if they aren't *your* sort of slave/Owner, it's just not going to work out. Compatibility first.

Once in a great while Joshua will act out, out of extreme stress and frustration, usually triggered by difficult outside pressures that have driven him to the end of his rope. When that happens, he's usually more dismayed than I am about five seconds after it's done, and feels terrible. I do what I can to alleviate whatever's driven him to such extremities, but we both understand that it's not cute, it's not funny, it's not tolerable, and it's not acceptable. It's an aberration that should be kept to an absolute minimum.

On the other hand, I think what some owners mean when they say that they don't want a "doormat" has nothing to do with obedience. I think what they mean is that they want a slave who is thoughtful and proactive, who is self-motivating; and requires very little attention and supervision. Sort of the opposite of "Which three eggs should I scramble, Master?" Instead, a slave who would get up before the owner, figure out by themselves (through experience) what the owner wants for breakfast, have it invisibly ready when the owner gets up, and expect no praise for it, being satisfied by the job well done and the fact that the owner deigned to eat it.

I'm often taken with the fact that one of the biggest complaints of slaves is that their owners don't pay enough attention to them, and expect them to maintain their slavery discipline, internally and externally, with less supervision and micromanaging and petting and punishing and tinkering and just general attention than the slave would like. In some cases, it's like the most abusive thing that the owner can do is to ignore them and watch TV, just expecting things to get done like an invisible and unthanked hotel staff! Yet owners who want that (even some of the time) are considered mean and abusive.

It's possible that "don't be a doormat" might be incoherent-owner for "Just bring me my damn dinner—no, I don't feel like deciding what, I'm hungry and you know what I like—and let me watch TV, and go entertain yourself, or do some virtuous activity, or clean the damn house—you know what needs doing!—and don't ask another bloody thing of me for tonight, just concentrate on my comfort, even if that means leaving me alone and not bothering me for orders or whatever, damn it! Use your damn brain to figure out what would be best for me, and motivate your damn self to do it without me having to bother with you. Good service should just appear out of nowhere and go away when I'm done with it!"

However, I've also seen dominants who say, "I like a feisty slave," and their submissive preens and then does some abominably bad behavior, or perhaps the two events are reversed and the statement is used as an excuse. What seems to be really going on there is that the dominant knows, on some level, that their control over their sub is tenuous at best, and it's a way of pretending that they don't mind it, and not looking at the fact that they might prefer them to be more obedient and well-behaved. There's not much that can be done about that situation, until the dominant decides to try for more control, and either get it or have it shoved in their face how little they actually have. Or, on yet another hand, the dominant might be a jerk who finds it amusing when their sub acts out and makes other people uncomfortable.

So it's a question of why they do it, and what secondary gains do they get from it? *Quo bene?* If the dominant doesn't mind it, or finds it entertaining, fine. If it's a problem, then the dominant needs to refrain from feeding the negative behavior. I'd say that if you want to punish brattiness, the best punishment is shunning or isolation in some way, taking attention further away from them. The point needs to be strongly made that it is a privilege to be here, and one dependent on the submissive's good behavior.

And honestly, although submissives constantly use the term "doormat" as a negative example of what their owner thankfully doesn't want them to be, I've never actually met a full-time consensual slave that I'd characterize by that term. Not one.

Q: What about Masters or Mistresses who don't let their slaves ask any questions or bring up anything negative at all?

Raven: To me, any owner/master/mistress who refuses to let their slave say anything negative, or complain at all, is using their slave as a tool to prop up their fragile egos and ensure that they never actually have to do any personal growth. I see it a lot, and it disgusts me. I mean, really, if you can't bear to hear gentle criticism from your *slave*, someone that you utterly own, who is totally vulnerable to you, what kind of a weakling are you? A friend of mine once commented that some (not all, just a certain percentage of wankers) would-be owners are trying to get slaves so that they will be protected from ever having to actually learn any relationship skills.

For myself, I'd rather hear a criticism from my slave than from anyone else. I know that he honestly does want things (and me) to be better, and that's his only agenda. I can't necessarily trust the agenda of outsiders, but if my boy gently points out that my fly is down, I know that he's not doing it to humiliate me but to keep me from getting humiliated by someone else.

The owner who won't listen when their slave is having a problem or is unhappy is like the car owner who refuses to pay any attention to that grinding noise coming from under the car every time you make a right turn ... until the U-joint fails and the driveshaft drops out on the road in the middle of the highway. (Happened once to someone's car and we all had to hitch a ride home.) If something's wrong, I want to know *all* about it, before it blows up in my face. Denial is *never* a good option. It's stupid.

To be fair, however, it is perfectly acceptable for the owner to mandate that the slave frame their criticisms in a respectful manner. If you're a dominant and you're having issues with your submissive's unfettered honesty, start with this:

1. Imagine your sub saying the worst opinion they've voiced yet. How could they have phrased it so that it would still be that opinion, but it wouldn't make you feel like they were undermining the dynamic? That's a fine line, and you can't allow yourself to err on the side of "feeling undermined"; there can't be censorship to spare your ego. But things can be said in a respectful manner. What's a respectful way for them to say things that are potentially hurtful to you? Figure out how your slave can phrase them in such a way that they sound earnest and respectful and honestly distressed, not contemptuous or nagging. That will take work on the part of both to figure out what words and tone and frequency is acceptable, but it could work out so long as the rules are not designed merely to shut the submissive up and keep the dominant from having to hear anything that might spoil their little fantasy.

2. What are the times and places for them to air their opinion? For instance, my boy is not allowed to criticize me in public, in front of other people. You might set aside time each day for them to air her opinions (in the manner laid out above), or perhaps have "formal" and "informal" times.

3. Remember that statements about their physical health, stress level, or emotions that are currently interfering with her ability to function are not opinions, they're valuable information that you need immediately, so that you can adjust your demands and expectations for the moment. So are things like "Sir, before you walk out the door, your shirt is on inside out," or "You're about to hit that dog! Stop!"

4. Now that you've figured out how and when they are allowed to voice their opinions, train them in this. That way

they are allowed full communication of all things in their head, but when they do it, they remember that they're still yours (because they're doing it in the way that you want them to) and it doesn't undermine the dynamic.

5. Now your end of the bargain is that as long as they say things in the way that you've taught them, you can't react badly. You're the owner, you have to be mature and accepting about all the shit that's in their head. You don't have to do what they tell you, but you can't react angrily and defensively. That can lead to them thinking you don't really want to know them unless they're perfect, and they'll start hiding parts of herself from you, and that way lies disaster.

Joshua: If even brief questions of clarification were not permitted? I imagine I'd find it very frustrating and pointless. I could likely phrase every question as a statement, possibly making heavy use of, "I do not understand your request." It is mostly pointless verbal gymnastics, though. "I don't know where the proper intersection is." "We have both wheat and rye bread." "The Safeway is closer than the Stop & Shop." I'm sure this would become irritating very quickly. Training the slave to communicate without making a pest of themselves is a more subtle process than "Don't question my orders."

On the other hand, if the relationship is not an intimate one, I think it can be appropriate for a master to severely restrict the submissive's free communication, especially if the slave is inclined to offer unwanted unsolicited opinions, criticism veiled as questions, and other obnoxious verbal habits. (I disagree with my master on this one.) In that case, I think it can be beneficial to require the slave to request permission to speak freely, at least until they learn how to regulate their speech.

Q: When I get PMS every month, I argue with my master. He normally doesn't have a problem with me expressing my feelings, but I just become terrible then! Should he tell me to

shut up for that whole week? Should I be trying to keep from him how I'm feeling about things?

Joshua: My master permits me to speak fairly freely and offer my opinions, disagree with him, and give constructive criticism in an appropriate and respectful way. While he values my opinions, I can be a whiny and argumentative bitch when I'm in a bad way. We've tried a few different things to keep this in check.

First, we came to an understanding that there is no real need for me to express my opinion on any subject more than once a day, if that, and that I ought to be able to sum up my opinion in a few brief sentences. (No coming back an hour later with, "...and another thing!") The first time I say something, it is information. The fifth time, it is just bitching. This was really useful for me.

We generally have a policy of completely brutal honesty with each other, but during a period when I was in a really bad way he restricted my ability to express my emotions freely to a specific daily (or near daily) situation. Since this is a recurring and predictable period of insanity, you might try giving your master a day's warning so he can temporarily suspend your right to speak freely. Mark it on his calendar. If during that time you have what you feel is legitimate criticism which you must tell him—and I know that in that headspace it *all* seems like vitally important and entirely legitimate criticism, even when tomorrow you might think that it's silly—you might consider doing it in writing.

It might also be useful to have a mandatory "cool-down" period between the time something vexes you and the time you are allowed to bring it up with your master. For some folks, this helps them gain perspective. Other folks just stew in it and get themselves all worked up, so it doesn't work for everyone. It may help to have something calming and/or distracting to do as a cool-down.

The best thing is to be able to maintain some awareness of how irrational you are at any given time, even if you can't stop it. Just say it, out loud, to your master. It can help if your master gives a set response to the hormonal behavior, rather than attempting to debate with you when you are in that state. You may deny up and down in the heat of the moment that this tear you are on has *anything* to do with your hormones, but if he won't engage in the argument it's like flinging yourself at a wall. Eventually, you get the point.

I know when I get all caught up in some emotion, part of me is standing back watching the carnage, helpless to stop the whole mess. I know I've said some terribly inappropriate things, followed in the same breath by, "Wow! That was inappropriate," and while I know that I intended to follow with an apology, what comes out is even more inappropriate than the first thing. It is like I can come up for air for just a second but then I get sucked right back down into it. It is incredibly frustrating.

After a while, I was able to occasionally say out loud that I was being irrational while we were in the argument. It wouldn't generally derail me though—I would say, "I'm being paranoid and irrational right now, but you are still wrong. And let me tell you why..." Baby steps, you know? But then he'd say, "Stop. You're not in a rational space, and I'm not going to talk about this until you're in a better place. Approach me about it tomorrow if you're feeling better." And that would be that. And isn't that the strangest thing? It is so nice to have someone just put an end to it.

Q: My master asks me what I want to do, and I just say, "I don't know." I can't tell my master the things that are really in my head. I don't think that those are the answers that he wants to hear.

Raven: Which is exactly the answer that he most needs to hear.

For my boy, I have him say, "I have no preference," but only if he really has no preference. It was difficult for him at first, because he feared that if he stated his preference, either I'd be angry at him, or else I'd just do that, and then I would be catering to his whims and not the other way around. Eventually he did become convinced that I asked in order to know, not in order to do that thing. If the choice is X or Y, and he prefers X while I prefer Y, then if I have that information I can decide whether to indulge him and do X, do X because I'm not strongly committed to Y and can afford to be generous, do Y while attempting to make it easier for him, or do Y and tell him to suck it up and deal. Whatever happens, it's still my judgment on the matter.

But by not telling me his preference, he robbed me of information I could use to fully and knowingly make choices. Of course, it also took a while for me to believe that he really does have little to no preference in many things. I am stubborn, opinionated, and extremely willful, and I have strong preferences on most things. He doesn't, and many of the ones he has are vague at best and easily overridden by seeing me made happy. But that was part of my really internalizing how opposite (and wonderfully complementary) we were in so many ways.

(Yeah, yeah, I know, it's obvious that we're really different. But people are raised to think, "You wouldn't like that done to you, so don't do it to others," when really we're too different for that kind of generalizing. So it took a while to quiet down the little voice that said, "He really likes that? Whoa! I would hate that! I would chew off a limb! I would kill myself or preferably someone else! How can he really like that!" Talking to other long-term slaves helped—"Yeah, you guys really do thrive in an environment that would drive me to violent insanity! Wow!")

If the dominant becomes angry after getting a respectful but honest answer from you, that's a problem ... and it's their problem. It's only yours in that you need to decide whether this relationship is a deal-breaker for you.

Q: My slave sometimes pushes me verbally, as if the intent is to make me blow up and hit them. Does my slave just need a takedown? Should I give it to them?

Raven: In the beginning of our relationship, Joshua did that a few times—tried to push my buttons in order to get a certain reaction, whether that was more attention, or more control, or whatever. Sometimes I think that it was only half-conscious on his part. I caught it, and called him on it—pointed out what he'd done, and why that was unacceptable to me, that it was manipulative and I wasn't interested in giving him a takedown. If he really felt that he needed a takedown, he could come to me on his knees, explain in depth his reasons for needing one, and beg for it. Maybe he'd get one, and maybe he wouldn't. And maybe he'd get one in a manner that he didn't expect.

He was chagrined—he'd been able to manipulate his last boyfriend just fine. He'd even manipulated him into being physically abusive, which then made him feel superior because he'd made the guy lose control. At any rate, after a few times trying this with me, he never did that again. Now when he wants attention of a certain kind, he comes and humbly asks for it. He also understands that he might not get it if I'm busy, and that's just too bad.

It's really on the dominant to make this one work. If the slave wants to help, they can tell the dominant the ways in which they were pushing the dominant's buttons in detail, so that they can put a stop to it the next time. They have to be able to catch it and call them on it, but not overreact and think the slave is doing that when they really are just tired and forgot something.

Q: What about submissives who really need a takedown to submit, whether physical or mental? What if they need it to feel like the dominant is really their superior, and thus worth serving?

Joshua: Some people need to be physically overpowered in order to fully submit. Some people can only submit to someone who is more clever than them, or more successful, or more insightful, or has better emotional control, or whatever. I think that which one they pick has a lot to do with the values and the (for lack of a better phrase) "conflict resolution tactics" they were raised with. If you are accustomed to disputes being settled by force, then it may be very difficult for you to fully submit to someone you could wrestle to the ground. If you are accustomed to people gaining favor or power by giving money and gifts, you may have a hard time fully submitting to someone who you give money to.

For me it is emotional control. If I can needle someone into losing their temper, I feel like I have control over them. It doesn't matter if they beat me up afterwards. In the early stages I would try to go at my master, and he wouldn't respond. I'd push harder, and he was immovable. It would end up with me suddenly realizing that I was acting like an errant toddler, and my master was calmly treating me like just that. It was very humbling, but it was also comforting to know that his impulse control was that good, and that no matter what I did he wasn't going to lose it.

On the flip side, if you have a slave who gets caught up in continual power struggles, it can be instructive to refuse to engage with them on the "battlefield" of their choice, even if you are confident you can win. If they get physically aggressive, don't knock them around or restrain them—don't even touch them. Tell them calmly and politely that they will sit down now. If you think they really need to be knocked around, get someone else to do it. If they are the type to try to lawyer their way out of rules or show how clever they are by proving you wrong, it can be better to smack them before they even finish their sentence and make no comment whatsoever on the merit of their arguments. Whichever way it goes, make it clear that their preferred method of resolving disputes is entirely irrelevant to this relationship. Make it clear that if they think they can retain power by being stronger than you (or more clever or whatever) they are mistaken. Make the only valid field of combat one where you have such a clear advantage that it would be pointless to challenge you.

Obviously, if there is any kind of a power struggle, a dominant should never engage their submissive on a front where they are at a disadvantage. Force them to engage with you in an area where you are confident you will win, or refuse to engage. (I've known dominants who will orchestrate situation without the submissive's knowledge to give themselves an unfair advantage, but I think that is problematic in a long-term relationship.) In any case, once the dynamic is well established, I don't think it matters so much.

Rights and Limits

Q: What do you mean that slaves don't have rights? Isn't a slave entitled to a few things, like respect and care?

Joshua: You are missing a key point here. There is a difference between what a slave is entitled to, and what a slave may be granted.

Let's say I walk out of my house and it is a lovely spring day. I enjoy that weather and I might even express how nice it would be to have more days like this. Does that mean I feel I am entitled to nice weather? If it is cold and wet tomorrow, am I going to feel like I've been mistreated or led astray? I am free to *feel* entitled to nice weather, for all the good it does me. The weather doesn't care. I can rail at the injustice of each stormy day and have a good sulk about it, but the weather does not ask my consent and is not moved by my arguments. So I take pleasure in the good days and I try to handle the bad days with grace. That is all I can do. To refuse the pleasure of the good days is needless martyrdom, which serves nothing but my ego. Accepting (and even enjoying) what your master chooses to give you is not the same as being entitled to it.

It's when a slave says "You are a bad master because you are not giving me X" that they express their feelings of entitlement. Not only that, but for a slave to claim that they deserve to be treated with respect (or compassion, or fairness) will almost certainly include the slave setting themselves as judge of what behaviors and attitudes demonstrate those things, and whether the master has met their standard. Few slaves would claim they deserve respect and then feel that condition was being satisfactorily met just because their master assured them they were respected. The entitled slave wants their master's actions to reflect what the slave believes is appropriate respectful behavior.

In reality, if the master actually believes that they are obligated by some moral standard to treat their slave with respect, it will be by their own definition. If the slave does not feel respected, that is the slave's failing, not the master's. Perhaps the master will care if the slave *feels* respected, perhaps not. If the master does care, they are better off adjusting the attitude of the slave than changing their own actions ... perhaps teaching the slave to feel respected by what is actually given, not what they think ought to be given.

One very controversial M/s website made a list of things that a slave is not entitled to, including such things as respect, loyalty, affection, compassion, appreciation, consistency, gratitude, explanations, or fidelity. What it *doesn't* say is that a master is not permitted to allow a slave these things. It doesn't even say that a slave oughtn't come to expect these things if they are given to him or her on a regular basis. It only says they have no inherent right to them. The slave has what rights the master grants them, not the rights the master (or the slave) thinks all slaves ought to have, or the rights that the master's other slave has, or the rights the slave was granted by a previous master, or the rights extended to slaves in a any given culture or popular work of fiction. The slave has the rights their master specifically chooses to extend to this slave in particular, for some period of time.

That's why all those months of preliminary negotiation are so important. They give the slave time to figure out if the rights that they will be granted are the rights that they want.

Q: How do you see the difference between what a slave is entitled to and what they need?

Raven: I own a car. Is it entitled to gas, oil, brake fluid, transmission fluid, and trips to the mechanic? Well, regardless, if it doesn't get those things, it won't go. This is maintenance. Maintenance is necessary, if annoying. Part of knowing your slave inside and out is knowing what they can't function well without, and what can be dispensed with, or allowed as a gift. This will vary from person to person.

Ideally, the owner shouldn't make that decision based in any way on whether this "need" is inconvenient to them, and would be so much simpler if it was classed as a "want" and possibly eliminated. Instead, they have to do the hard work of teasing apart the slave's emotions, associations, and motivations around the subject in order to make the most objective decision possible. This is one of the hardest discernments to make in M/s. It's not easy, and it may not get easier over time. First, the slave probably isn't objective about the subject. There are a lot of things that we strongly desire that we could probably survive without, and we'd get over the emotional trauma of not having them in much shorter order than we believe. There are probably also things that we are dependent on, and could be trained off of with time and patience, but they certainly feel like a need the first moment we lose them. Then there are things that it would really leave lasting scars, or possibly destroy trust, to have to give up. How you determine which is which in the face of the slave's tear-streaked face begging, "Please don't take that away from me, I'll go insane, I need that, I really do," is a delicate game.

But in the end, if the owner gets it wrong, reality will win out. If the slave is ordered by the master to clearly articulate their needs, and the master has enough power and authority over them to make them do so, and the slave does it, and the master ignores it, and things go terribly wrong...

...then it's on the master. Their fault, their responsibility, their bomb. Why? Because it is the master's opinion of reality that counts in Making This Whole Thing Work. They're in charge. That means that their take on it counts, in the sense that it's the one that gets followed. If you're really in charge, it's all on your head. If it's not all on your head, then you're not really in charge.

That's why this isn't work for every bozo who wants things his own way.

Q: Can't a slave have limits?

Raven: Before I speak to our admittedly anomalous situation, let me say that limits are something that should be discussed in depth at the beginning of any potential D/s or M/s venture. I'll say right up front that it's the submissive's job—and right— to decide where the lines get drawn in the beginning. That can include saying, "I won't give myself to a dominant who doesn't hold these particular limits," and it probably should start out that way regardless of where it goes. It can also include saying, "I agree to let my owner decide where the limits are." This, however, should only be done once trust is fully established, the relationship's boundaries are clear, and it's certain that both parties are fully committed to mindful deep enslavement.

Given that: In our relationship, Joshua doesn't have limits. I have the limits. Limits are my job.

This is in sharp contrast to SM play, where the top makes the rules but the bottom sets the limits. That's as it should be in that situation. With dominants and voluntary submissives, they share the setting of limits and come to a compromise. With full enslavement, the owner holds the limits for both parties. Of course, Joshua is with me because he inspected my limits, and decided that he was fine with them, way back in the beginning many years ago. Eventually he gave up the ability to enforce his limits.

Note my use of the word *enforce*. It doesn't mean, nor imply, that he does not have things that he cannot physically or psychologically do. He certainly does, but it is *my* limits that keep me from asking for those things (because I know him well and I want him to run at optimum speed). Since he has become psychologically "leashed" to the point where he cannot consciously disobey me (which we'll discuss further in the Internal Enslavement section), that means that it's all on me to make sure that the limits that are enforced between us are healthy ones.

Whenever he tells people that he has no limits, many of them will jump to the same conclusion. "Of course you have limits! You just think you don't! What if your master told you to..." (add heinous crime of your choice). So what does it technically mean when we say that?

1. Obviously, he has physical limits. If I ask him to flap his arms and fly, or even benchpress 400 pounds, that's not going to happen.

2. There are things that I could ask him to do that he would be psychologically unable to do. For example, if I told him to take a hatchet and hack up a mutual friend of ours, while he might pick up the hatchet and start towards them (perhaps after gods-know-how-much begging and pleading to rescind the order) with full intent to carry out that order, I doubt that he would be able to make himself do it, because he's a nonviolent little sissy who's never raised a hand to anyone. Maybe, if I was standing there yelling at him the whole time in command voice, pushing him verbally ... maybe. Not likely, but maybe. But that would be more about him utterly surrendering to my will and going into some sort of fugue state where he simply reacted to my orders like an automaton. So that's also a limit. I consider it in the same boat that I consider the physical limits—in other words, not part of what we mean when we say "no limits". If you could not manage to do it on your own—not *would not*, but *could not*—it's the same thing. Doesn't count.

3. What if I asked him to do something that he would be able to manage psychologically, but would have extreme objections to—like put poison in someone's teacup, or molest a child, or stand there quietly while I hacked off his finger? Would he do it, if I ordered it? Yes, he would. No question. He might argue, he might beg, but if push came to shove, he'd do it. Feeling horrible, perhaps, but he'd do it. Of course, he'd be a wreck afterwards, and I'd be in karmic trouble so deep that I ... am not even going to think about that.

So that's where we start defining "no limits". It isn't as though those things aren't "limits" in his head, in the sense of "the boundary beyond which he desperately does not wish to go, and/or believes is a very bad idea to cross". It's that he has given up the ability to enforce those limits in any way, and so he might as well, for all *practical* purposes, not have them.

Some of you are probably thinking now, "Why would anyone be so moronic as to put themselves in a situation where they became psychologically incapable of saying no to someone else, even if they ordered you to do something like that?" If you feel that way, then you shouldn't be in a Total Power Exchange or Internal Enslavement relationship, and that's perfectly OK. (As to why someone would willingly do it, again, that's in the chapter on IE.) But if you intend to get into something like that, or even a relationship that has the distinct potential to *become* a TPE or IE relationship, you need to make damn sure beforehand that that this individual will be safe to do that with. You should *not* feel OK about surrendering because you feel like the dominant will respect "your" limits, even when you don't have the ability to enforce them any more. You should only surrender if you are entirely certain that these are limits that they hold *in and of themselves*, that they would hold anyway.

It should not be a matter of saying, "Please, Sir/Ma'am, don't ever hurt me in this way," and them graciously agreeing not to do so, because they love you or are feeling generous or whatever. It's a matter of them saying, "Well, of course not. I wouldn't ever do that sort of thing. It goes against my code." Which means that they need to have a code *already in place* that you agree with totally. They need to prove to you by their actions that they *actually hold to it all the time*, even when it's difficult to do so, and that you are not just believing that of them because you're head over heels crazy with adoration. (Having a third party that you trust to interview them helps. The best test, however, is time and observation.)

One thing that we did was to put in an insanity clause. For me to order Joshua to do the things I've mentioned above, I would have to have cracked. Gone stark raving nuts. Assuming that he would still be alive 24 hours after I'd lost it entirely, he is under orders to get away from me and go somewhere safe immediately that I show behavior so far off my code that I would need to be demented to evidence it. That's not his limit. It's mine. It's part of why he trusted me that much. Seriously, think about such a clause in your agreements. Slaves need to be that careful. They are that vulnerable.

(No, I have no history of mental illness, and this is not us preparing for an actual potential problem. However, one never knows what might happen; some friends I know have developed sudden temporary mental problems from bad reactions to new medications. And anyway, putting it in is the right thing to do.)

Joshua: I don't have limits. My master has the limits. I have no say in them. He does to me what his honor and common sense will allow. Of course, if he wasn't an honorable and sensible man, I wouldn't have been fool enough to let myself get enslaved by him. I came close to doing that sort of thing when I was a teenager, and I learned my lesson. Thankfully, that first experience was short-lived, and the man was inexperienced and had enough mixed feelings about the whole enslavement thing that he never took all that firm a hold of me. I intentionally crossed him on something big, and he let me go.

In contrast, a dear friend of my master got herself deeply enslaved by a real jerk who had little regard for her well-being, and that was by all measures a profoundly abusive relationship. After a few years, he told her he no longer wanted her and without any warning or explanation he left her on a street corner downtown. I don't believe she ever saw him again. Looking back on those situations, both she and I have a hard time emotionally believing that our former masters did anything "wrong". We both felt—and still feel—that they didn't "violate our rights". They were just unpleasant and unfortunate situations, and we'd rather not do that again, if at all possible. Intellectually, we both know that it was wrong and would be advising others in that place to leave, but emotionally it still feels like they had the right to do that. This is another reason why submissives who have the potential to become deeply enslaved need to be careful who they choose. If we sound like a broken record on that one, there's a reason.

When I first started out with my master, he put down three hard limits that he didn't have to—that he would not interfere with my school and work, that he would not take my money, and that he would not (beyond safe sex and bloodplay) restrict my sexual or sadomasochistic activities with the three individuals who I had been involved with at the time we took up together. I laughed a little at this, and told him that while I entirely understood why he felt more comfortable with these limitations in place, that there would come a time when they'd be irrelevant. It wasn't that I was telling him he was wrong to want these limits; I just had a strong idea that our power dynamic would progress far deeper than he was (at that time) willing to let himself hope was possible.

I was right. It is one of the very few things with him that I can say that about. By the time he formally accepted me into his service, it would have seemed ridiculous to the both of us to include limits of that sort. We have a contract, because he loves putting agreements in writing, but it basically outlines his expectations of me and the ways in which his ethics do and do not permit him to treat me. It was for me, more than anything else, an informed consent agreement. I swore an oath to say that I knew exactly what I was getting into, and intended to do everything I could to live up to his expectations.

Q: How can you tell the difference between someone who's being abused and someone who's just the slave in a really intense TPE dynamic?

Raven: I think that the first question you need to ask is: why are you asking this? What's your motivation in trying to figure out someone else's dynamic? Do you believe that you have the ability and the moral right to interfere if it doesn't measure up in your head? Think carefully about why you're judging before you start judging, because your motivations will affect your judgment. So will your ability to get past projecting your own likes and dislikes on others.

I think that the first thing to look at is whether the slave is happy, contented, and fulfilled. Is their self-esteem good? Has being a slave improved it? Look at that before you look at the activities that they're doing. Of course, this does mean that you have to actually take the slave's word for it, but if you think about it, to do otherwise is to insult their judgment in a way that does not see them as a competent, independent adult peer. (Which is something you may already be mentally accusing their owner of doing.) If they honestly tell you that this is the life they want, you have to accept it, at least as far as your interactions with them go. If they are unhappy and their self-esteem is suffering, that's a warning sign.

Joshua: I really don't like this idea that the more intense a TPE relationship is, the more it resembles abuse. A TPE relationship with an agreeable submissive and a reasonable dominant will not generally look abusive to people who know them well, no matter how intense the power exchange is. A lower-intensity D/s relationship where the submissive is struggling with basic obedience tends to look more abusive, because the submissive seems to be continually being told to do things they don't want to do.

For a TPE relationship, many of the control-oriented things that would be abusive in a supposedly egalitarian relationship are just the way that these two people prefer to structure their lives. Comparing the type of control in a healthy TPE relationship to the type of control in an abusive relationship is similar to comparing SM to assault. A behavior that looks very abusive from the outside might be a behavior that the eager submissive has been begging the dominant to do for months. Don't be so quick to judge.

It reminds me of a scene I watched in a public play space, where a submissive was getting worked over very hard and was very sincerely begging the dominant to stop. Someone approached the host and suggested he should intervene. The host pointed out that the submissive wasn't restrained in any way and could easily step out of range of the dominant's blows. The submissive showed no inclination to actually get away, despite their protests. That was clear consent, no matter what it looked like to the casual observer. It is likely that if someone had tried to interfere, the submissive would have been just as irritated as the dominant.

If you *are* going to look at the activities, ask yourself how you'd react if this person (or someone like them) was deciding to do this thing entirely of their own free will. Would you feel like you had to prevent them from doing it to themselves? People in the BDSM scene (and the rest of society) choose to do all sorts of strange things. Just because you wouldn't like it doesn't mean they don't.

The owner makes them eat from a dog bowl and keeps them in a cage? Reasonable adults in the BDSM scene beg to be treated like puppies and kept in cages. The owner wants them to get breast implants or reduction? Reasonable adult women choose this for themselves all the time. The owner wants to tattoo "Master Bruce's Bitch" across the slave's ass? You may think that's inadvisable, but otherwise reasonable people choose to get inadvisable tattoos all the time. But a slave getting "Master Bruce's Bitch" tattooed across their forehead would cross that line in almost any community.

I realize that line is very subjective, but many people are quick to insist that anyone who does something they themselves would find terrible could not possibly be sane and reasonable. If it seems to be working for the people involved, leave them alone. The next time someone tells you your sexual activities are the product of a deranged and troubled mind, remember what that feels like.

On the other hand, I have to point out that a relationship doesn't have to be "abusive" to be bad for you. I spent five years in a volatile, violent (and egalitarian) relationship where I sometimes wondered if I was being abused, and sometimes wondered if I was abusing my partner. I eventually figured out that I didn't have to prove a case of abuse either way to decide that this was just bad for both of us, and I should get the hell out. If you really want to leave, it doesn't matter if it's abusive or not. Something is clearly wrong.

Q: Can someone be fully enslaved if they have children (who have to come before the master) or if they have a job (which takes them away from their master)?

Raven: That's a difficult question, and one which there's been a lot of argument over. It's true that the feeling of enslavement has to go both ways. Just as the owner's hold over the slave can slip if things go wrong, the owner's feeling of being in control can also slip due to outside circumstances. I'm not ready to say that anything that limits the owner's wishes even a teensy bit will automatically make the slave unenslaved. If the owner has a strong need to be able to beat and torture their slave on a public street corner, and is limited by the fact that they live in a society that will arrest you for that, it doesn't make the slave unenslaved. Or, rather, it doesn't have to. (If such necessary thwarting makes the owner feel threatened, that's a dominant with a lot of problems and one hopes that they actually haven't enslaved anyone.)

It's more of a gradual slippery slope. Each outwardly-imposed limitation which interferes with the needs of that particular owner does gradually eat away at the feeling of enslavement on both sides. At some point, that does cross a line, and the owner feels like they really don't have sufficient authority over the situation to make it feel like ownership. I've struggled with things on the edge of that line, and I've had to jettison and veto things that might pull it over. Of course, the key words here are *the needs of that particular owner*—in other words, what gets in the way of satisfaction for any given owner. What annoys the fuck out of one owner doesn't matter a damn to another one.

I'll use children as an example, since you've brought it up. For some male masters, being able to knock your female slave up, breed her like livestock, see her squeeze out the fruit of your precious genetic seed (a need just as atavistic and primal for some men as making babies is for some women) and then knowing that she is slaving over your rotten little clones, that can be a satisfaction great enough to more than offset the fact that she is changing the diapers rather than giving you an on-demand blowjob. For others, a squalling brat would be just something that got in the way of the slave giving the owner their total and complete attention. (I'm deliberately using coarse language to describe the far ends of both situations.) There's a whole continuum in the middle of dominants who see a submissive raising their children as a useful and important service, or who had children before they discovered D/s and are doing their best with the situation until the kids are gone, seeing it as an outside influence that neither has much choice about, and must wait out.

For myself (and here I will get personal) I've been a single parent and raised a child. I am now done with that. At this time in my life I would find that the responsibilities of a slave's child would interfere too much with my priorities, and trigger my own personal sense of what annoys me. So, no, for purely personal reasons, I am 95% unlikely to take on a slave with a rug rat in tow. That's my personal preference. It might not be that of another potential owner.

What about that final 5% chance? I've thought about that. There is an exceedingly tiny chance that I might become extremely attached *to the child*. It's unlikely, but within the cosmic realm of possibility. So what then? I've loved, been devoted to, and raised a child before. If I felt that way about the child of a putative slave, then I would give them a choice: either we'd agree it still wouldn't work, and bid a fond adieu ... or I would take over full responsibility for that child. *Full* responsibility. It would become my child in every way, including legally. The slave parent would be in every way a full-time nanny for *my* child. I would make all decisions, and that child would become as much of a priority for me as my own child was when I raised her. My slave would simply be my support in doing so, and as such would be the one to do the menial parts of parenting while I did the important ones. It would be the same as when I tell my boy that my job is a higher priority than he is, and that I expect a big part of his job to be helping me with that job.

Before all the married heterosexual submissive women with children run screaming (well, actually, it's fine if you run screaming, I'm not heterosexual, not shopping and wouldn't be right for you anyway), I would ask that people try to understand why this would be the only ethical way that I, personally, could see to do it. If I did it that way, then it wouldn't be a horrid and continual inconvenience thrust upon me. It would be my own choice, my own project, and no one else's. (Someone else might make a different choice, from different values.) But, again, this is only a tiny likelihood, as I am happy to be child-free.

Let's use a different inconvenience to contrast. Some owners would find a slave working a job to be a horrid inconvenience that would make interfere with their priorities, and their sense of control. For them, the feeling of mastery means a stay-at-home slave who is always there on demand, no matter when they get home. OK, fine. For me, while a 60-hour-a-week hard-driving career would be a problem, a flexible 20-hour-a-week job doesn't annoy me very much, and the benefit of my boy handing over a paycheck to me to contribute to household expenses is a far greater satisfaction. It doesn't make either of us feel like his control is slipping, and he's still quite enslaved. It's a matter of the owner in question figuring out where that line of annoyance and lack of feeling control is, and not moving over it. Enslavement is a matter of mutual perception and emotion, which often has little to do with objective reality. In fact, it's really a mind-over-matter sort of thing.

And there is *nothing wrong* with a dominant saying, "If my slave does XYZ, that will cross the line for me, so I won't take any slaves who must do XYZ." That's just being honest about your needs, and heading off future drama. For example, there are slaves out there with specific mental illnesses that I wouldn't take on—not because they aren't worthy people, or couldn't be good slaves for the right master, but because *for me*, it would feel like the illness was in control of them, not me. It would quickly cross my line. To send such a submissive away would be a kindness to both of us; they would need to find someone for whom that doesn't cross the line.

There's also the issue of immediate versus delayed gratification, another intensely personal issue. To give a personal example, as I write this particular answer, my boy is currently in school. It is fucking inconvenient. It does interfere. Sometimes it sucks. Sometimes it comes perilously close to that line. Why don't I tell him to quit? Well, for one thing, I picked out the schools, the degrees and certifications, the career path, and sent him in the first place. I chose that training on the basis of what would serve me in the future, part of my overall long-term plan for crafting Raven's perfect slaveboy. And, unfortunately, I cannot order him to become a certified massage therapist, complementary health care worker, Asian bodyworker, and Shiatsu practitioner, while sitting chained in my living room. (It'd be cool if I could pull that off, but it's not possible.) I decided on what I wanted him to be, set the priorities, assessed the risks—including the risk to my convenience—and decided that short-term interference was worth long-term gain. I am definitely seeing it pay off as he goes through school. Like child-raising, I also know that school will eventually be over, but the rewards will remain.

Another owner might assess the risks, and say, "Nope. Not worth it," and that, too, is fine. Much of ownership is risk assessment—about your slave's mental and physical health, about what makes them feel enslaved, about what makes you feel like you're still in charge. (And oh, boy, is it not fun when those last two things clash ... but that's a different problem.) That line will vary depending on who you are, and no owner can make that decision for another one. Although they can say, "I wouldn't do that. But hey, it's your life."

Q: My new master wants a contract but I don't. I don't think that we need one. Do we?

Raven: A contract is useful for many people because it spells things out. If both people work on it together, then it's a way of making sure that you both have the same expectations, the same definitions, so that later no one says, "But I didn't think that you meant *that*!" All relationships have boundaries, and it can be both enlightening and comforting to have them spelled out. Also, it's a bonding activity.

To the submissive who feels that contracts are unnecessary: It's not your call. If they make your putative dominant feel more secure, then you should go along with it happily. Indeed, the fact that he's the sort that would want a contract says something about him: perhaps he likes to have things spelled out, likes to know where things stand at all times, dislikes open-ended boundaryless feel-as-you-go situations. This is something that you're going to have to learn to love and appreciate, or at least work with, in him. You'd best start with this contract.

I'm the sort who loves a contract too. (Ours is in the back of this book, for your perusal.) And those things, above, are true for me as well. I hate situations where everyone just sits around assuming that everyone else is on the same page, and everyone just waits to see how it all turns out. I like boundaries. If someone wanted to be in a service relationship with me, and they objected to a contract (not just shrugged and said, "OK, it isn't usually my thing but whatever you want, I'll go with it," but actually objected), I would be suspicious. I would wonder what fire they didn't want their feet held to on a later date, as it were.

Q: Do you allow your slave to vote in elections?

Raven: I know M/s couples where the slave isn't allowed to vote, because in the master's mind only free people vote, even if the slave's lack of freedom isn't recognized by anyone but them. I also know couples where the owner lets the slave do whatever they want with their vote. I take a somewhat more practical view.

One of the things that I use Joshua for, and certainly one of the things that I get a *huge* amount of flak for from people who don't understand deep consensual slavery, is his vote. I am an activist, and I am a very politically aware person, and I have a vested interest in voting going the way I want it. His vote is a resource for me to use, just like his hands, his paycheck, his genitals, and his computer skills. So when elections come around, he asks me how he should vote, and then he votes that way.

I have had M/s people who also confiscate their property's paycheck get all weird when I said that. Something about voting seems ... off limits, I suppose. I've also had kinky friends get upset because it seemed "unfair"—I had two votes when they only had one. Oh well. Too bad. Get yer own slave.

To be completely fair, if he had serious moral reservations about the way that I wanted him to vote, and he begged me to be allowed to vote for some particular person or rule, I would take that into consideration (and probably let him). However, he's totally not interested in politics, to the point where he won't be in the room when my wife is watching the news. So his vote is just another thing that would be wasted if I didn't use it.

Q: My master hates my family, and wants to forbid me and the kids from seeing them. I know that they have problems, and they've said rude things, and been kind of mean, but I really want to keep seeing them, and I think that the kids ought to see their grandparents. Does he have the right to stop us? Do you stop Joshua from seeing his family?

Raven: I think it largely depends on why your master wants to cut them out of everyone's life. If he sees them treating you (and him, and the kids) badly and with disrespect, if he sees you falling into old patterns of codependence and placating them when you're with them, if he honestly thinks that these are not role models that he wants for his children, then you had better trust his judgment or go back to a more egalitarian dynamic where you can make your own mistakes and he has no say.

I don't have any technical control over my wife, but I declared her father to be *persona non grata*, because he's an abusive dickhead. The one time he came to our place, he insulted everyone and expected to be placated, and she fell back into going along with it. I won't play that game. I said that while she can go where she likes and visit whom she likes, he wasn't coming onto our property again, and I wasn't ever going to deal with him. She agreed to that, because she knows that she could ask the same of me if she really hated someone that I was bringing over. If she'd been my sub, it would have been a complete cut-off, period. We don't have kids together, but if we did I would find them a different grandfather.

As for my boy ... him I do have the final say over. His family disowned him for a while because of his lifestyle choices (many of which involved moving up here to live with me), so I said fine, they were out of his life. When his mom began to make overtures of reconciliation, I agreed to let him see her (and stepdad and siblings) once a year for a few days, but only if they were decent to him. He has orders to walk out if they are mean to him. He isn't allowed to associate with the nasty uncles and grandpa who send him abusive, hateful emails. He isn't even allowed to read the emails—I read and delete them, because they distress him so much. If he's visiting his mom and those family members show up and begin to behave badly to him, he is to leave immediately without speaking to them. I am not interested in mean people abusing someone who is my responsibility, and making him feel bad.

Not all families are nice. Many of them suck. Many of them would help you, but only at the cost of your self-esteem. I think that a reasonable owner wouldn't limit contact with a reasonable family, but the problem is when the dominant honestly thinks that the sub is better off without them, and the sub doesn't agree. It can be really hard for an adult with emotionally abusive parents, with whom they have a lifetime of codependent behavior, to see that and realize that they need to separate for their own growth and mental health. Sometimes it takes an outside party to say, "This isn't healthy. You need to get away from them." The difference is that if the outside party owns you, they can enforce that. (And if the dominant thinks that it's unhealthy for the sub, I can well see how they might think it unhealthy for the kids to be around such people, and to see their parent become codependent around such abuse.)

So let's put it this way: If your master ordered you to confront your parents and say, "Mom, Dad, if you want to see me and the kids ever again, you're going to have to stop Behavior XYZ around us, period," ... would you? If not, he's not in charge. They are. You're letting them have more authority than him. They still own you, when push comes to shove. Maybe he doesn't like that. Can you blame him?

(And if you did say that and *they* wouldn't respect it, then my dear, they aren't worth it.)

So if he really thinks that it's bad for you and the kids, then you need to take a long hard look at how you sacrifice for them, and who really owns you.

Q: What areas of Joshua's life does Raven control?

Raven: All money is mine, including what he earns. I say where it gets put. He pays the bills, on my instructions. If he wants to buy something bigger than a small lunch or the equivalent, he asks permission. All his clothes are authorized by me. He has his uniforms—winter, summer, formal, fetish—and work clothes for grubby jobs, his yoga clothes, and some "normal" outfits for work. Every day, his doings revolve around what I think he ought to be doing that day. We generally start the morning, before even getting out of bed, with a discussion of the day's tasks.

He may have what friends he likes, but what he is allowed to talk about with them is restricted. I control how he is to treat my wife, my friends, my co-workers, and my clients. Anyone can email him, though. I control how he is to behave in public—and that means anyone besides me being present.

The opposite side of this is that he has no control over anything that I do, in any part of my life, or who I do it with. If there are things in his life that I am not controlling, it's generally because I really don't give a damn about them. I don't care when he goes to the bathroom, for example, or what sort of shoelaces he wears.

Every dominant is going to have a different list of things they're interested in controlling. Some will want to know every time their submissive goes to the bathroom; others will let their subs have any kind of sex with anyone they like. Some will want to have a say in their career and others ignore the entire issue. Some will want to pick out clothes or design a diet, others won't be interested. Some slaves are allowed high-powered jobs that fly them all over the country, and others aren't allowed out of the house. It is extremely variable, and my overview above (as well as Joshua's more specific list below) are not meant to be anything more than interesting examples, not be-all and end-all. A sub can guarantee, though, that sooner or later a dominant will probably start to control something that they really don't want to give up control over, and that's when the real submission starts.

In his answer to this question, Joshua was allowed to pick out some of the everyday rules he's required to live under. You'll notice that they aren't sexy rules. In fact, many of them might seem like small things that it's silly to even legislate, but we're including them anyway. It doesn't always occur to a beginning dominant that if some little thing that a sub does (or forgets to do) continually annoys them, they can make a rule about it, no matter how small it is. Learning to be an organized dominant starts with getting a clear picture of how you'd like things to run, and setting up the rules to reinforce that ideal.

Joshua: I am under a broad set of rules regarding obedience, personal access, appropriate conduct, and the right stewardship of my master's possessions (including myself). The general overview rules are listed in our contract, in the back of the book. They have only rarely needed to be altered.

The more specific day-to-day rules of practical household behavior are in a file my Master sometimes refers to as The Rulebook, and they get changed periodically if circumstances change, although most are standard long-term rules. I'll include a selection of these here for interest, as the whole thing would be too long and boring to include. Any of these rules can be changed, modified, or overridden by my master, without giving reason. Granting exemptions does not invalidate the rule in future situations, no matter how frequently exemptions are granted.

> *Life1: Joshua may not be submissive to anyone else to the depth that he is submissive to Raven. He is a privately owned slave, not a public utility. Giving that*

to anyone else cheapens it. He is to behave courteously to everyone else, but that is all.

Life2: Joshua may not commit suicide. His life and death are not his to choose.

Work3: When Raven is utterly immersed in work to the exclusion of all else, Joshua is to do the following:
    a) Never take it personally. It is never about anything but the work.
    b) Unless other appointments call, stay within calling range, but find virtuous work to do.
    c) If no assignments have been given, and Raven seems too busy to provide one, and there is nothing currently awaiting doing, then find what entertainment you will.
    d) If Raven emerges, offer him food. If he declines, remember rule a).

Work4: Joshua is to make it easy for Raven to know what Joshua's schedule is at all times. He is to update whatever method is decided on, promptly and at least twice a week. Raven will endeavor to remind Joshua of his activities for the next day, and will take those activities into account when deciding on Joshua's bedtime. All errands must be authorized by Raven. If Joshua is out and discovers that he will be significantly late getting back, he must call and let Raven know.

Work6: When Joshua has finished any given order or chore in the house, he is to come to Raven for further orders. He may not wander off and choose his own activities unless he has prior explicit permission from Raven. If Raven is busy with something (like guests in another part of the house, or working), or if he is not home and Joshua is, Joshua's priorities should be:

a) homework

b) any list of items that Raven has left

c) his own devices

Joshua may not indulge in any of the latter until the former two are entirely finished. The only exceptions must be verbally granted by Raven.

Work8: When Raven comes to check on Joshua and asks for a status report, Joshua should give him the following information, as clearly and concisely as possible:

a) What he is doing now.

b) How important he feels that activity is.

c) How long the activity will take to finish, as best he can estimate.

d) If it will take longer than a quarter hour, when the next stopping point will be.

Example A: "I'm paying the credit card bill. It really needs to get done. It will take maybe twenty minutes, and there's no good stopping point, unless it's an emergency."

Example B: "I'm playing a game. I could stop in about five more minutes without losing my place. It's not important, but I'd really like to be able to play at least half an hour if that's possible."

Health4: Approved doctor-prescribed medication must be taken as directed. Approved over-the-counter drugs and herbs can be taken at Joshua's own discretion, provided the intent is not recreation, especially with regard to herbs tinctured in alcohol, and any psychoactive or stimulant herbs.

Health6: No dusting or vacuuming without permission. (Josh's Note: I'm allergic to dust! Hard for a houseboy, eh?) Joshua is to stop as soon as he notices any *asthmatic symptom, even if it is not a convenient stopping point. He is not permitted to independently choose to do anything that he knows sets off his asthma or any breathing-related or systemic allergies. He is of no use to his master if he is in bed running a fever all day.*

Health8: Joshua may not have any derivative of sugar cane, or high fructose corn syrup, except for very small negotiated amounts in substantial meal-type food, such as sweet sauces on meats. Real maple syrup, honey, fructose, and fruit juice concentrate are permitted. Absolutely no aspartame or saccharine, in any quantity. Malitol is acceptable in small quantities, sucrolose and Ace K in very small quantities. No caffeinated or decaffeinated drinks.

Service1: On trips with Raven, Joshua is to be in charge of making sure that the car is in good shape for traveling, the baggage gets packed in the car and transferred in and out of the hotel room, that Raven has adequate correct food and drink, that Raven's medications are packed and easy to find, that Joshua's own meds are packed, that the toiletries are packed (including a hairbrush), and that Raven has the materials necessary to give his classes. (This latter must be ascertained by asking.) He is in charge of finding restaurants, gas stations, laundry facilities, and running emergency errands. If camping, he is in charge of the kitchen and all food prep. If there is shamanic work to be done, he is to follow orders and mind all physical objects. Non-shamanic physical objects are entirely his responsibility. Shamanic physical objects are only his responsibility if Raven entrusts them to him for a short time.

Service2: If Raven and Joshua are eating a meal together, Joshua is to make sure Raven's needs for food and drink are taken care of before he tends to his own. Joshua is ideally to bring Raven a beverage before serving food, or at the least the beverage should be served with the food.

Companionship3: When Joshua comes home, he is to seek out Raven, and offer him affection and signs of devotion. If Raven is seated in a non-public area, he is to kneel and put his head in Raven's lap.

Travel1: Joshua is to drive in ways that do not upset Raven, even when Raven is not in the car. He must keep at least one hand on the steering wheel at all times when driving. Knees are not appropriate substitutes. If Raven clutches the dashboard or warns him of an oncoming car, he is not to take it personally.

Sex3: While solo masturbation is allowed, Joshua cannot waste all morning jerking off. He may not give himself an orgasm without Raven's presence and permission. He can play with his junk, but all orgasms come from Raven.

Sex4: After Joshua gives Raven an orgasm or is allowed to have one, he is to thank Raven for allowing him to do so.

Communication3: Joshua must make eye contact when apologizing for anything.

Communication4: In general, Joshua is not to speak to Raven in a disrespectful tone. What constitutes a disrespectful, overly sharp, or otherwise bitchy tone is entirely up to Raven. If Raven dislikes his tone, Joshua *must modify it even if he disagrees with Raven's analysis. If Joshua feels especially indignant over Raven telling him to modify his tone, he should take that as a warning sign and consider whether that feeling is an indication of the sort of mood that makes him prone to disrespectful behavior.*

Q: Do you control Joshua's Internet time?

Raven: Joshua's internet rules are these:

❖ May not dick around on the computer when other chores I have specifically asked of him that day remain undone, unless I grant him down time.

❖ May not dick around on the computer if there is actual computer work to be done.

❖ May not start drama on any forum.

❖ May not respond to any drama in any way that might feed it.

❖ Any post that makes him feel a surge of righteousness during writing must be checked by me for snarkiness, inappropriateness, or general nastiness, and edited or canned if necessary.

❖ Online journals are Evil (they all too often foment drama and allow people to indulge passive-aggressive behaviors), and may only be used for posting announcements, recipes, or other innocuous and non-drama-creating, non-whiny information. Online journals of people who use them to indulge in the former unpleasant behaviors are off limits.

❖ Any Internet activity that threatens to take up far too much of his time will be eliminated.

❖ Any discussion list that makes him continually shake his angry little fists will be eliminated.

❖ Posting something angry, discourteous, or overwrought will result in being barred from that thread/subject.

❖ Internet privileges can be removed at any time for overuse or misuse. If it begins to take up too much time, it's out for a while.

❖ No discussion of me or my habits online without my permission.

❖ Spelling, grammar, and syntax must be as correct as possible. (One of the hard parts of being owned by a professional editor!) No slashed caps, no decapitalizing his name or pronoun, no cutesie internet writing customs, no "LOL", none of that. Correct English only.

❖ In general, Joshua is to behave with faultless courtesy when online, so as not to shame his master. His behavior as my property reflects on me, even in vanilla fora, and he is to remember that at all times.

Q: But what if he gets into an online argument and he's right, but the other person is misunderstanding him, and he really wants to say his piece? Is it fair to remove him?

Raven: This has happened, more than once. In each case, I removed my boy from the thread, stepped in, politely informed the individual who was negatively misconstruing things that I had removed him and his voice, and briefly explained why. In every case so far, the posters were so horrified that Joshua had been banned from that thread and prevented from arguing his point (a fate worse than death in their minds, apparently) by his Cruel Owner that they apologized profusely for getting him into trouble and dropped the whole thing.

Works for me.

Joshua: Regarding the issue of having one's words misconstrued, I will say that one of the most valuable things I've learned in service is to assess the actual importance of me being right and/or being seen as right in any given situation. Being allowed to express my opinion to all who will hear it and convincing people that I am right is not generally a top priority for me. If we're doing activist or educational work it is important, but then it is just a job. We are passionate about it, but there isn't a huge emotional investment in it on a personal level.

If you have a solid center and feel deep sense of purpose in your life, then what random folks think of your behavior becomes largely irrelevant. I act rightly in accordance with what I believe and the rules I live by. If someone I barely know chooses to think ill of me, there is little reason for me to care unless they have some kind of real power over me or intent to do me harm.

Trappings

Q: Who should be naked, the owner or the slave? Is nudity more vulnerable (in which case it's a slave thing) or the opposite?

Raven: I'm in the very odd position of having a slave who generally wears more clothing than I do. I very much like being able to be naked or nearly so in my own home. As I am fat, well-padded, well-insulated, and extremely cold-hardy (Polar Bear Club type) I'm fine with wearing nothing but socks or slippers in January, in a house warmed only by a woodstove. In fact, that's my dress code at the moment. (And besides, I have such a thick pelt of body hair that people have commented that I look clothed even when I'm not.)

However, my boy is usually clothed. There are two reasons for this. First, he's a skinny little thing and gets cold much easier than I do. Second, there's an interesting psychological aspect that has come up. Before I owned him, he was very much a slut and a whore, giving himself freely and fairly indiscriminately to all and sundry; his only limits were safe sex. He did sex work and porn, and for him nudity was a way to advertise his lack of boundaries. (No boundaries, no standards; he's the sort that really needs a short leash, and to be kept off the street.) However, once he was owned by me—and suddenly he couldn't touch anyone without my permission, and my rules keep everything between his legs for myself—a change occurred. He began to want to dress more modestly, especially around other people—the people to whom he could no longer offer himself.

Some dominants find that they have a rather modest submissive on their hands, perhaps one who was raised with rules about what sort of clothing was appropriate for the "right" sort of people, and forcing them to be nude (or nude except for "socially inappropriate" clothing) is a powerful act of attitude-changing. A dominant can use nudity as a way to force them to be constantly aware of their slavehood, and the lack of access that they have to ordinary free-person privileges such as standard clothing. In these cases, the dominant remaining clothed reinforces that they are free, and thus makes the submissive vulnerable in comparison. (A dominant can also keep them nude or scantily clad because they like the look of it, of course.)

But I discovered that for Joshua, it is being covered up that reminds him best that his body now belongs to me, and is to be exposed only for me and my pleasure. If we go to a play party, he is locked into an obscuring chastity harness. No strangers will ever view his bits unless I am there to show them off. This means that me being nude has become my right to do what I want with my body, and his being clothed (unless I order him to take his clothes off) means that he has no such right. It also echoes the fact that I can have sex with whomever I want (given the polyamory limitations negotiated by myself and my wife) and he can't. So he doesn't walk around naked in front of people any more outside of our house, and generally I never order him to take his clothes off unless I want him to get into bed with me.

So it's been interesting to turn this nude little slut-boy into an almost Victorianly proper modest serving-man. And, ironically, it adds to my feelings of possessiveness. So whether the slave should be naked depends on the dominant's preferences, and the slave's mindset.

Q: What about clothing and uniforms? I'd like a uniform, or at least I'd like my M to tell me what I ought to wear, but so far there's been no interest. How do I spark interest in this?

Raven: I went through this with Joshua. He really wanted to wear things that he knew I liked, but it wasn't a high priority on my list—there were behaviors that were much more important to get right as far as I was concerned—and frankly I wasn't sure what I wanted, as far as everyday clothes.

Finally, he asked for a uniform, something for him to wear every day so he wouldn't have to worry about clothing choices. (Clothing choices, in general, worry him; he would rather not bother.) He asked me to decide on what it should be. Confronted with this task, I suddenly discovered that I had a whole lot of preferences. If I was going to have to see him in the same thing every bloody day, it was going to be something that I'd want to look at.

So ... colors are a good place to start. I like earth tones, so Josh's uniform is brown and green and rust and gold. (Maybe you could start by asking your master what colors he likes to see, in general—and then don't bitch if he chooses ones that you don't like to wear, or don't personally think that you look good in.) I decided on brown Dickies pants or shorts (and we discovered that Dickies classic pants really show off a nice ass), dark green band-collared long-sleeve shirts or dark green sleeveless T-shirts (the latter shows off his nice definition), and vests in rusts, browns, and golds. The winter uniform does tend to look like that of a hotel waiter, but that's life.

Point is that I had a lot more preferences than I thought, I just had to sit down and put it together. But I also had to consider the overall look. This is my property; what do I want people to see when they look at him? Because that's going to reflect on me. Sometimes I see dominants who let their crotches rather than their common sense rule these choices. It's one thing to have your submissive dressed like a whore in the house; quite another in the grocery store. Even if you dig the idea of "using" the hapless onlookers as part of your humiliation scene, it's not fair to the onlookers to be so used without regard for consent. (It's also gotten people arrested, and resulted in the dominant having to bail out the tearful and angry sub.) At the very least, do your submissive and the public a favor and have a "public" version of their "uniform", however you conceive of that, which is not too revealing or obscene. They can always change as soon as they get home.

Slave clothing doesn't have to be sexually obvious to be submissive, anyway. There are various sorts of outfits that say "service", from the plain housemaid's dress to the modern low-grade service uniform, which seems to have become a polo shirt with logo and khakis or black pants. Some leather houses have taken on the polo shirt as their house uniform, complete with house logo, but their subs tend to be mistaken for employees in the CVS or Target. (Which, perhaps, is its own humiliation and reminder of their position.) If you want to dress your slave up strikingly in public instead of making them inconspicuous, remember that stylish draws more admiration (for your property, for you as their partner, and for your sense of taste and character) than slutty. It's also less likely to get anyone in trouble.

Joshua: It may be a matter of mentioning the criteria by which you choose something to your disinterested dominant, and seeing if you at least get an "OK, sure," out of them. This can be like: "I always pick dish detergent on the basis of what's cheapest and doesn't smell too strongly; is this OK?" or for clothes: "I tend to go for casual stretchy things in jewel tones; do you like the way that looks, or do you like it when I wear the long flowing stuff like this dress?" Giving the owner a menu of choices that they can comment on, if only obliquely, can help. So can periodically asking, "Do you like this outfit?" and paying attention to when it's "Yeah, it's OK," and "That one's really nice." After you get a few extra-positive responses, compare them and see what they have in common. (This is part of the sub's task of closely observing and noting what the dominant likes, without bothering them about it unduly.) Then you can note that they like short skirts, or blue, or whatever, and wear that.

Q: What about haircuts and hair styling? I'm scared of the idea that my mistress might make me shave my head.

Raven: Hair is one of the big ways in which people express their identities, and it's often one of the first and most classic ways that a master or mistress takes ownership of a slave. Some will simply order them to get a different haircut, one that the M-type prefers. Some will make a big deal of removing all the hair from the entire body, either to remain that way as a symbol of submission, or to grow back in a new style. Since hair does regrow, it's a good way to drive home that change of identity with a method that's repairable if the relationship doesn't work out.

When my boy came to me, he had a mohawk. Since his teens he'd had all sorts of weird hairstyles, shaved head, mohawk, crew cut, half-shaved with spikes, and almost always some odd color. His hair was the way that he showed his individuality, mostly with punky hairstyles.

Well, there's no way to recover gracefully from a mohawk (and it was a bad 'hawk, too) so I had it shaved off. He was just fine with that—liked the military look of a shaved head. I don't. So from that time on—and that was six years ago—I decided that he would never cut his hair again, or style it in any way more complex than a ponytail or single braid down the back, and it would remain his natural chestnut color. Oh, he hated that! He begged me periodically to let him shave his head again, until it became obvious that it wasn't going to happen. It got in the way, it required fussing with, it wasn't utilitarian. But it was awfully pretty, and I liked it, and that's enough, right? And it makes a great handle to put him on his knees.

Actually, he still hates it, and he'd shave bald in a second, gladly, if I let him. But every time it gets in the way, or that he has to braid it or fuss with it, even if he wishes with all his might that he could cut it, it's a reminder that he can't ... because it belongs to me. Long and straight is the one hairstyle that he never wanted—his punk friends associated it with hippies—and now he's got it, because I like it aesthetically. I think there's actually something more powerful about "This is done because my owner finds it appealing, and my feelings on the matter are entirely irrelevant," much more so even than "This is something that my owner is doing to me in order to prove a point or break me further." In other words, sometimes the most powerful thing is the thing done not at all for the slave, but entirely for the master's whim.

Q: Should the owner pick a name for the slave? What if it's an awful or humiliating name?

Raven: Naming is a very powerful thing. It defines who you are in many ways, and to rename someone is to change them in some way. I think that it's important for the dominant to know well what the connotation of a particular name is *to the submissive* before you tack it on to them. If you decide that she's going to be Buffy, and (unbeknownst to you) her immediate connotation is the horrid, stuck-up girl named Buffy who she hated from the third grade, that might have repercussions in her actions once she's internalized that she is now Buffy. If you've decided that he is to be named Cocksucker, well, what does that entail to him? Maybe you think it's fun and humiliating, but does it mean that he thinks that's all he's good for? Humiliating names are especially tricky, because what is humiliating is intensely personal and subject to many shades of connotation.

Objectifying names have similar issues, but they often have "job" associations. Make sure that the job you name the slave is the job that you want them to Be—not have, Be. Because that's what you're asking of them. Make sure that it's not so specific that it forces them into too narrow a mold. I formally named Joshua Raven's Boy, with the intent that this title would be wide enough to encompass all sorts of things.

Joshua: I remember watching a scene in a historical movie where a lady got a new maid. She asked the maid her name, and the maid said "Isabella" or something similar. The lady said, "Isabella? That is no name for a maid! You'll be Mary from now on." I also remember a bit from a very dry old book on service in Victorian England where it mentions some folks always calling their cook Susan and their gardener Thomas and so on, because that was the name of the first person who'd held the position and they can't be bothered to keep track. I really had to laugh thinking of that one, because I am the seventh person my partner has named "Raven's Boy", which is hardly even a name to begin with.

Q: What if I want my slave to use third-person speech? Can that work well?

Raven: You need to ask yourself *why* you want your slave to use third person speech. Some slaves do, some don't, depending on what their owners want. Generally I've found that the two main reasons the owners command it are: A) personal pleasure—it makes them hot to hear it, or it gives them warm fuzzies to hear it; and/or B) it's done as a mindfulness exercise, to reinforce that no part of their life will now be "normal" and free. Decide why you want it, and make your slave aware of those reasons. When they do it right for a period of time, reward them, if only with an approving word. When they miss, calmly go back to "Rephrase that." But the positive reinforcement is important.

Joshua: I think that the key to graceful third-person speech is to not refer to yourself very often. Starting every sentence with "This slave..." seems to go against the point of the exercise. Use passive voice whenever you can—instead of "I washed the dishes," or "This slave washed the dishes," say "The dishes have been washed." Talk about yourself less. In a high-protocol situation, which is what is likely if there's third person speech going on, there is often little call for it. In fact, talk less in general. Speak only when spoken to, and say only what needs to be said. Before you say something, think: "What value does this information have to my dominant?"

Service Vs. Control

Q: What's more important to slaves—the need to serve, or the need to be controlled? And what about dominants? What do they want most?

Raven: That depends entirely on the individual involved. Obviously there's a continuum between the two, and control-oriented subs will often be expected to give good service, while service-oriented subs will usually be expected to submit to control. (And mind you, disclaimer, disclaimer, I am not intending to say that either end of that spectrum is better, worse, healthier, more slavey, whatever. None of that. All good, just different, every combination thereupon wonderful in its own way, and that's good because different M-types want different things! There, disclaimer over.)

Just from watching the demographics, I estimate that there are more control-oriented submissives than service-oriented ones. But that may just be what I've seen swim by. It could also be that for those whose primary drive is for service, there are areas of life which might satisfy that urge enough to not make slavery a first choice, whereas control-oriented subs might more quickly come to a point where it's consensual slavery, abuse, or a cult.

I'll let Joshua speak to the continuums of submissives, as I already talked about the celebrity/parental continuum of dominants.

Joshua: I'm a service-oriented slave, which means that I find service more rewarding than being controlled. The M/s aspects of control are very enjoyable for me, but they aren't an end unto themselves. Using control to further service makes sense to me; there is a purpose to it. Without service, what is the purpose? To demonstrate that the dominant has control over me? In a serious M/s relationship, I would want that to be a given, not the primary focus.

If the purpose is to entertain the dominant with feelings of being in control, that makes me a little nervous. People who make their own essentially-purposeless entertainment their primary focus are not the sort of people I want to spend the rest of my life with. Besides, in my personal experience with dominants like that, I've found they get bored easily. They are always after something better, something new, something more extreme. They seem jaded and eventually lose interest in the supposed entertainment. That isn't a situation I want to be in.

On the other hand, control is the main motivation for some slaves. They want to feel held, taken, wrapped up in the will of someone else. It makes them feel safe, or desired, or sexy, or devoted, or pliantly selfless, or all of the above. Service, when it's given, is just one more way in which they are controlled. And, of course, there are dominants on both sides.

Q: What happens when the dominant and submissive have opposite needs on this continuum?

Joshua: It can be extremely frustrating to be a service-oriented individual with a dominant who is only in it for control (just as the opposite can also be true). In a relationship with a control-oriented dominant, there are often extended periods of "training", with either no end goal, or an impossibly high end goal. This is very frustrating to a service-oriented sub, whose self-esteem is often strongly based in their ability to meet (or even exceed) their dominant's goals. By their perception, they are constantly in a state of failure. Continual micromanagement and correction, rather than being comfortable, can become an ongoing reminder of this. Desperation for praise and success can lead to unhealthy (and perhaps self-harming) behavior.

To remain healthy, a service-oriented sub in this position must recognize that the master wants the struggle, and that "excelling" in service to this type of master means trying your best, letting them see you struggle, and showing emotional resilience when faced with the (perhaps) inevitable failure. In my experience, a self-aware service-oriented sub may get to the point where they no longer struggle. They see the futility in it, and simply do as they are told to the best of their ability, accepting success and failure with dispassionate grace. While this can be a life-changing and transcendent epiphany for the submissive, it may lead the control-oriented master to lose interest in them.

With a less perceptive master and a more casual relationship, the submissive may find that enacting that struggle beautifully is the best service they can offer. Another possibility is that they accept that their only service to that master is entertainment and emotional gratification, but if this is to be at all satisfying to the submissive, it is best when it is discussed up front, and less perceptive masters may not think to do this.

Control-oriented subs are in an equally difficult situation when they end up with a master who prefers service and is less interested in control for its own sake. Once they become skilled at performing the services that the dominant wants, the dominant may slack off and no longer correct constantly, assuming that the sub will just continue to follow the rules and find gratification in doing so. This makes the submissive feel as if there is not enough control, and that they are not really being dominated any more. They may feel that they are being taken advantage of, and that their master is not a "real dominant". They may (intentionally or unintentionally) undermine their training and act out in order to receive correction.

For the control-oriented sub in this position, they can either internalize the dominant's "voice" so thoroughly that they make themselves feel controlled even when the dominant is not paying attention to them, or they will need to leave ... or the dominant has to step up the level of everyday control.

All this simply underlines the fact that people need to thoroughly compare expectations and assumptions before they commit to a relationship. I see the desire to be controlled and the desire to render service to be entirely independent variables. For someone who is equally motivated in both, the distinction is largely irrelevant, because they are unlikely to run into these kinds of incompatibility. The distinction becomes useful when dealing with someone who is much more strongly motivated in one but not the other, because they often don't appreciate that the other motivation can be just as meaningful to a different person.

Q: What's the motivation behind the urge to service?

Joshua: I tend to group service motivation into three categories: transactional, devotional, and positional. *(This will be explicated further in Joshua's future book, Real Service.)* A transactional motivation is when the individual is serving because they are getting an equal exchange out of it. This would include the waiter and the cleaning lady, who are getting paid in money. It would also include "I do this for you now because I know that you'll do that for me later, so it's worth it." It's good for every power dynamic to include at least a small amount of transactional motivation, because it keeps people in touch with their needs, and noticing whether those needs are actually getting met. However, while this can work very well for short-term encounters, the constant accounting gets tricky when it's every minute of every day. Eventually someone thinks they are being short-changed. Transactional motivation will only go so far, also, because it is easily swayed by personal desires and selfishness.

Devotional motivation is when the submissive serves out of love. The dominant is the most wonderful person in the world, and they gain satisfaction from helping this object of their loving feelings. Love is an amazingly strong motivation, and can carry someone a long way in the face of difficulty. The drawbacks to this category is that on days when they don't feel all that loving—which inevitably happens, we're human and we piss each other off—they may not feel like rendering much in the way of service, either. A submissive motivated primarily by devotion would do well to cultivate a little of the other two types of motivation to pull them through the "I hate you today" mornings.

Positional motivation is when the submissive serves because it is part of their identity. They take pride in serving as perfectly as possible, and they are the ones who get up to help because it needs doing, regardless of who is asking. They are the most likely to attempt to cultivate "pure" service, treating it as an art and requiring little in the way of appreciation. On the other hand, they are also the ones who are most easily taken advantage of by unscrupulous people who want something for nothing. Putting the chairs away after the PTA meeting for the fiftieth time won't work for the transactionally-motivated submissive ("What's in it for me?") or the devotionally-motivated submissive ("I don't love you; why should I do what you say?"), but the positionally-motivated submissive will get up and do it anyway, because it's their very identity.

This category is the "ideal" slave in Laura Antoniou's *Marketplace* series, where slaves are sold to random wealthy masters who may or may not be even remotely worthy as people, and the slaves are expected to serve their monied masters to the best of their ability anyway. However, in real life another drawback of positional motivation is that it does tend to objectify dominants and perhaps see them as interchangeable, and the slave's own specific master may want to be seen as a little more special than this. Adding a bit of devotion to the mix will help in that regard, and cultivating some transactional motivations will help keep the submissive from being taken advantage of too often.

Q: My master doesn't seem to want to do anything to help me feel like a slave. He just wants me to bring him dinner and then get out of the way and clean the house while he watches TV. This is not sexy! I feel more like a maid than a slave.

Joshua: I think it is very important to get a clear idea of how much importance your master places on training as opposed to simple obedience and service. I am speaking from experience here; I was severely chastised a year or so after moving in with my master for complaining that he wasn't being appropriately domly, and insisting that if only he'd put more effort into disciplining me then I wouldn't be having such trouble.

In the beginning of the relationship he did more formal protocol, but that tapered off, and it wasn't because he'd lost interest or become lazy. This was his first real enslavement-type relationship, rather than a simple D/s relationship, and eventually he realized that *for him* the main function of the BDSM training and discipline was keeping the slave interested. In the long run, he didn't find it an effective or desirable way to secure obedience or improve service. For him, it was a lot of work for little reward; he didn't enjoy it and saw no reason to continue it. He expected me to obey when I wasn't being entertained or sexually aroused.

I struggled against this terribly, but eventually I came to understand it—not when I was chastised, though. At that point I only understood that my behavior would not be tolerated. It took another year or more to really come to understand and accept what my role is. There was no easy way to it; it was just a matter of time and doing the work—not the mental gymnastics of trying to feel more enslaved, but the actual day-to-day service. Just keep doing the work and keep acting the part and it'll come.

You feel more like a maid than a slave? Good. Then you're getting somewhere useful. (If you feel more like a girlfriend or housewife than a slave, that's a much harder place to move beyond.) It might be useful to think of it as primarily being your job, rather than primarily being a source of emotional fulfillment. Your job can and almost certainly will provide great emotional fulfillment, but on the days when it doesn't, you just do your job.

I don't mean this to sound depressing; it's actually intended as encouragement and reassurance. Even if you aren't "feeling it", so long as you are doing your job, you are not in error and there is no need to feel guilty. Besides, feeling bad about not feeling the "right way" isn't going to get you any closer to where you want to be. Feeling confident and satisfied in the services you provide will, in time, help get you there.

Q: What about proactive, anticipatory service? I know that some dominants like it and others don't—but what happens when the sub assumes the wrong thing and misses? Isn't that a problem?

Raven: I *like* anticipatory service ... when it's done right, of course, which is the trick of it. I like it when within fifteen minutes after I start coughing while absorbed in my work, a cup of hot herbal tea materializes by my elbow. I like having my dinner appear, and knowing that it's something that I will like, because Joshua knows my tastes and isn't going to serve me okra or Brussels sprouts. I like it when something gets done for me in a way that I've never actually given an order about, but that is exactly what I would have wanted had I thought through and given an order.

I don't just like it because it's convenient, although the luxury of convenience is wonderful. It means that Joshua is actually focused on me, actually bothering to spend effort and attention figuring out ways to please me—and, more important, that he's actually seeing *me* and not some dominant icon in his head with my face on it. He's serving the person, not the office. That means a lot to me. Among other things, it means that this dynamic is working well and things are as they should be.

I'm willing to put up with occasional misses, because when he gets it right on it's really good. So when he misses, I simply correct his information. He's smart enough not to try anticipatory service in situations where there is both vague information and possible bad repercussions for failure (like wasting a lot of my money or time), and he does frequently ask me things like "Would you like this? Is that interesting to you?"

On the other hand, I did learn from experience that if the dominant wants proactive service as opposed to reactive obedience, it's even more important to put all the rules in writing, including their exceptions. If the submissive is going to have a long leash and less supervision, and will be expected to obey the dominant's wishes anyway, they'd better have something very specific to refer to when the dominant isn't around to ask. For reactive service, this is much less of an issue; if the submissive is going to be (fairly to completely) micromanaged and need only concentrate on obeying the order of the moment, then really there only needs to be one rule: Do What I Say. To put them in perspective, reactive service is Do What I Say, while proactive service is Do What I Want.

Joshua: In many ways I'm even more service-oriented than I am submissive. I find service inherently fulfilling even in the absence of strict obedience, and I would have a great deal of difficulty in a role where I wasn't expected to provide any meaningful service, no matter how much submission was involved.

It is interesting that "thoughtless obedience" is often listed as one of the characteristics of complete submission. My master has specifically held me back from thoughtless obedience, for his own reasons. I believe my master prefers … what is a good phrase for it … "critical obedience"? (Well, I am certainly critical!) What I mean is that he'd rather not have to ensure that all orders he gives can be followed out to the letter without thought or modification. If I'm in the middle of something and he says, "Josh, go do X", I'm not expected to obey without any thought. I am supposed to give some thought as to what he hopes to achieve with X and how doing X will affect the task at hand, and determine how best to meet my master's goals. If I have information as to why X might be ill-advised, or if the task at hand is in a more critical state than he might have realized, I am expected to say so.

As a trivial example ... before I met my current master, I was conditioned to drop to my knees at a certain cue. This was done at a level of near-thoughtless obedience. If I was, for instance, holding a pot of scalding hot water, I'd likely only dip down a little and then carefully set down the pot before getting all the way down, but that small reflexive dip could well be enough to splash scalding water on me. Having that level of reflexive, literal obedience means that the dominant needs to be very, very careful with their orders. By holding me back from that deeper level of reflexive, unthinking obedience, my master leaves himself the freedom to give less precise orders.

Q: I was at a leather conference, and in the cafeteria I saw a lot of paired-up D/s couples, each with their own tray. In no case were any of the subs waiting on the dominants. So I sat down and had my sub wait on me, because that's the way we do it, but we were the only ones at first ... until some of the dominants saw us, and handed their trays to their subs and sat down themselves. Isn't this kind of service just part of being a slave?

Raven: And that's exactly what we do, even in vanilla situations where there's a cafeteria line—I find a seat and he brings me food. Which includes, for him, buttonholing food prep people and finding out what's in the food, as I have allergies and dietary problems. Part of why I like to be served is that I suffer from hypoglycemia, and when I have low blood sugar, all food looks bad, even though I have to eat it or get worse. Making decisions about food is hellish for me in that state, and if I'm forced to do it myself, I've been known to say, "Oh, screw it," and either eat the first thing I see or walk away and get worse. So if we go to a buffet-type situation and I immediately sit down and say, "Get me food," he knows to just go and pick out something for me that is safe, and that he knows I like to eat, and get it in front of me as fast as possible. I may not even notice what it is until after I've eaten enough to get my brain back on line.

Sometimes I'll get in line, but that's usually when I'm in a good way blood-sugar-wise and there are many interesting things I'd like to check out. Then he follows with my plate, and gets what I point to. We return to the table, he puts down my plate and goes back for his own while I eat.

On the other hand, if I've been to this buffet four times this weekend (because it's a conference or something) I already figured out what was up there the first time, and I see no reason to go up again. I'll sometimes catch him studying my plate when I'm somewhere for the first time, to see what I chose, and then he'll be able to say the next day, "Do you want some of those little cakes again?"

It's not perfectly or exactly like this every time, because one has to adjust one's protocol to the particular situation. Public eating venues differ, and it's hard when there are dietary issues involved. (I'm allergic to, among other things, soy products. You can imagine how treacherous that makes the food industry for me.) If he doesn't know what I want to do, he watches for cues. If I clearly don't know what I want to do, he has instructions to make specific suggestions.

However, on the other side of things, I have noticed that some dominants (especially in America) are uncomfortable with too much hand-and-foot service. This seems to be because their image of themselves as strong and dominant is wound up with qualities such as "independence" and "self-sufficiency", and if they sent their slave to do every little thing they might look lazy or weak. This is especially prevalent with the ones who have a very protective Daddy-type relationship with their precious subs, rather than a "you're my tool and I will use you" relationship.

Me, I'd love to have a whole team of slaves to cater to my every whim. Not because I'm lazy, but because I have so much to do, and think of what I could get done with that!

Q: Well, I tried to do this with my dom, and he didn't want it!

Raven: Ah, there's always some form of service that the slave would love to shower the M-type with, and the M-type is like, "Get that away from me!" That's just personal idiosyncrasies. Service is never the same across the board.

Q: I want to improve my service to my owner, but I have so little time with my job, and I'm trying so hard, and still so many things slip by me!

Joshua: Talk to him about *his* priorities. Lay out your schedule for him, and make a list of the things you *are* doing, and the things you think you ought to be doing that you are not. Include a rough estimate of how much time you spend (or would spend) on each of these things. Ask him how important each of these things is to him. You might be disappointed to see some services you want desperately to be able to provide, very far down on the list or crossed off entirely. (I know I was.) Then again, you might be relieved. As slaves, I think we often value different things than our owners, and can have a hard time understanding their priorities.

You might also talk to your master about your financial situation and your work schedule. It might not be practical to cut back your hours at work or change jobs, but sometimes looking honestly at what your options are can make you more confident that what you are doing is the right thing. Depending on your budget, you can discuss the possibility of using higher cost, lower effort ways of getting things done. (For instance, we have a service in my area that will deliver your groceries. You could hire a cleaning service or lawn service. You can order out rather than cook.)

If you are his slave, all of your time is his resource, to do with as he sees fit. It isn't just your "free" time you give to your master. It is every moment, and every action. As a reasonable and responsible adult, he's going to allocate time for childcare, work, and so forth. He doesn't need to schedule you to the minute or address every detail, but if you are feeling a conflict in your priorities, that is something he *should* address.

Please keep in mind that "trying harder" is not a successful time management strategy. You are likely already trying harder. Effective time management requires looking at how much time and effort things *actually* take, not how long you'd like them to take. If you are overwhelmed and frantic, your master may be able to provide a much needed reality check here. He may also put a higher priority on your physical and mental well-being than you do. Overwork and high stress lead to illness and increasingly poor performance.

I know that as slaves we often want to be able to make things perfect for our masters in every way, but you are not an infinite resource. It is up to your master to decide how he wants to use you, and you need to give him all the information possible to make that decision.

Q: Have you found that service supports control, or undermines it?

Raven: Both, in different ways. It establishes control, in that giving Joshua (a very positional sub) a specific venue in which to serve binds him firmly to that venue. Being my boy is validating to his identity as a service-oriented submissive. It gives him a strong sense of purpose, a surety of knowing he is doing exactly what he's supposed to be doing with his life.

It diminishes control in that I require his service to be extremely (some would say unusually) proactive, and done gracefully with very little management from me, for the most part. This means that he has to have a daily level of lack of feedback from me that wouldn't work for a slave with a higher need for control.

Not that he doesn't need control. He does. He likes to be told what to do. But the way my life works, I generally have to run him right up there on the line with just barely enough feedback to keep him feeling enslaved. As he's gotten better and more used to it, I've moved that line further and further away. Every little thing that becomes unquestioningly natural for him helps to hold that line strong even as I move it. I think of him as a well-trained falcon who doesn't even need to be hooded or jessed any more, and will sit patiently on one's shoulder until told to fly at that thing, and will go off and collect it faithfully, and come back and deposit it and wait for his bite ... who can be out of sight, flying through the air, impossible for the owner to catch if he wanted it to, but the falcon would never think of doing anything but doing what he was told and coming right back.

Internal Enslavement

Q: So what is this Internal Enslavement stuff anyway? Is it the same thing as Total Power Exchange?

Joshua: The term "Internal Enslavement" was coined by Tanos, a slave-owner in the UK who founded the website *The Slave Register*. According to him, Internal Enslavement is "both a process and a set of practical techniques which use detailed examination of a slave's thoughts, emotions and past experiences to establish and maintain a solid and inescapable state of ownership. This is achieved through control of the slave's psychological states, in contrast to external enslavement, which is made inescapable by physical forces rather than the slave's internal psychological state. Legally or socially enforced slavery is an example of external enslavement."

The current accepted definition of Total Power Exchange, coined by Steven S. Davis in the mid-1990's, is "a relationship in which no impediment to the exercise of the owner's power is accepted ... Such things as safewords, contracts, negotiated limits, and anything else which recognizes, acknowledges, or formalizes limits on the owner's power are inimical to TPE."

The difference between these two terms is one of specificity. Total Power Exchange is just what it says it is: a (usually 24/7 live-in) M/s relationship in which one person has given all authority over to the other one. But it is still an umbrella term, and under that strict definition, there can be a lot of leeway. While the early proponents of TPE felt that the definition didn't count unless it was a live-in 24/7 relationship, later D/s folk adapted it to cover part-time relationships, as long as the TPE model stood whenever the people in question were together. It also leaves open the question as to whether the submissive in question is a voluntary submissive ("Every day I have the choice as to whether I leave this relationship, and I choose to stay..."), an honor-bound submissive ("I could theoretically leave, but I've promised to stay..."), or a psychologically bound slave ("I can't leave, because I can't bring myself to disobey any more...").

Internal Enslavement, on the other hand, is more specific. It is a system whereby the slave is slowly conditioned into a state where they are psychologically unable to disobey. This is done with their consent, and is usually an open collusion between both parties.

Q: Isn't internal enslavement just a form of brainwashing? Isn't that wrong?

Raven: Ah, we've actually braved the evil word "brainwashing"! That's an awful way to put it, and it's likely one that will make people wince, but it's pretty right on. (I've seen reams of writing that detail specious and desperate reasons as to why calling it brainwashing isn't accurate. As someone who's actually been doing it, it looks like brainwashing to me, sorry.) What I've done to him—with his consent and collusion—is indeed a form of ongoing mental conditioning. It is geared toward, and has so far been very successful at, creating such mental blocks in his mind that he is unable to disobey me in any way. Not physically unable, but mentally unable. You can do that to people, if you do it right—and if they are suggestible sorts, which I think may be the key. The more naturally suggestible that someone is, the better this works.

This is a scary thing. I think that people who react badly to slaves talking about how "they have no choice" are probably seriously repelled (frightened, disgusted, whatever) by the very idea. Something in their head says, "This is wrong. To do this to another person is wrong (or dangerous, or whatever)." Sometimes that thought process then becomes "...so I refuse to believe that it's possible, because then I would think much worse of these people, and especially their owners." Sometimes they're just skeptical about whether it can be done at all. Either way, I think that's where these arguments come from.

I'm talking about slowly, carefully inducing mental blocks in someone until their body and their will simply mutinies and will not respond when they attempt to be disobedient. I mean inducing something in someone so, as one slave put it, they could sit and stare at the suitcase, but would be mentally unable to actually pack it and leave. If you don't think that it can be done, I suggest doing some research on hypnotism, on trance states, on the sort of brainwashing that cults do. You may be surprised what can be done to a human mind.

Of course, in the latter cases, it's not actually done with initial informed consent. In our case, Joshua first agreed to serve me, thus giving revocable consent. Then, when we'd been together a year and he noticed himself start to have physical and mental resistance to any form of disobedience to me, we seriously discussed whether we wanted to move forward or back in this direction. He consented—which he didn't have to do, but he did it. That was the last independently revocable decision that he ever made, because after that we started the conditioning in earnest.

This is relationship built on a very different foundation from one that is fully or even partly egalitarian. In an egalitarian relationship, one of the basic rules is "It's wrong to try to make your lover change. While you can fairly ask them to alter behaviors if those behaviors don't affect their identity, you need to be able to love them for who they are and not ask them to become someone else." In M/s, that rule is cast aside. The whole purpose of "training" is to change the submissive's behavior, sometimes drastically. In internal enslavement, you can change them on an even deeper level. One of the crucial jobs of the dominant is to ascertain, objectively and realistically, what parts of them can be changed and what parts are immovable.

What makes this ethical is that: A) they signed up for it and theoretically knew what they were getting into; B) both people agree that the way in which the slave is being changed is for the better; and C) the slave has chosen as their owner a human being with exceptional morals, ethics, and compassion whom the slave has decided would be utterly trustworthy with their helplessness. This last one is crucially important, and really puts the initial burden on the slave to take the utmost care with their choice. More on that in other chapters.

We found, after a while, that if it was done right it didn't matter if he consciously wanted very much not to do what I wanted. The ideal is a slave who, when told to stand there and not move, even when they desperately want to move (perhaps they are arachnophobic and a spider is purposefully walking toward them) will stand there motionless, perhaps screaming, "No! I want to move! I need to run away!" and trying with all their might to move, but their body entirely betrays them and refuses to respond, even in the midst of terror.

Another example might be a slave who, whenever they contemplate doing something that they desperately want to do, but are strictly forbidden to do, simply becomes nauseous and headachy, and the more they contemplate it, the worse it gets, until they have to quit. Or, even better, every time they think about doing the forbidden thing, their attention just gets suddenly distracted and diverted to something else. "Gee, I wish that I could ... Hey, look, the stove needs cleaning!"

Does this leave the slave open to neverending abuse? I won't say that it's not possible, if the slave has chosen badly and the master/mistress is not a responsible and ethical human being. It may well use the same pathways as "battered spouse syndrome", only without the battering and the trauma. It's not something that any slave should give that final consent to unless they are dead certain of their owner (and ideally have been with them for a long time). I would never put down someone who wanted to keep that last outpost of "If things get bad, I can leave." That's perfectly reasonable. Obviously, most D/s couples aren't going to mess around with this. For one, thing, the dominant needs to know how to do it safely. For another, the sub needs to be fine with the idea. That's a rare thing, and so it should be.

For those who are already horrified by the idea, well, let's just say that I thought very long and hard about it, and about the ethics of it, before I started implementing it. As far as I'm concerned, I am a sane, rational, and non-abusive person. It's not just my slave who says so. I have never had a lover who claimed that I was unsafe in any way, or injuriously irresponsible. So I think that I can be trusted with that kind of power over someone. You, whoever you are, may not agree, but then you weren't the person who gave it up to me.

I can see why it would look frightening from the outside. Why, just think of all the ways that could go horribly wrong! Who could ever trust anyone that much? Who could ever be worthy of that kind of trust? Isn't this all too dangerous? Except that some of us are doing it anyway, and so far, at least in my house, it's working fine. Yes, I could be just brainwashing Joshua into thinking everything's OK when in actuality he's horribly abused. And really, there's no way to prove that conclusively unless you wanted to come camp out on my couch for a week and watch, and my wife would definitely have something to say about that. But I don't think that anyone who's met him could possibly mistake him for a miserable and abused human being.

Joshua: Entering into service, I was very clear that I was here by choice. I did not like the term "slave" because it implied I was held by force, and I was not. I was an honor-bound servant. Eventually, my master and I began to realize that he had increasingly reliable and effective control over me that was not dependent on my willing participation. I generally think of it as brainwashing, but I know that is a problematic term for many folks. To call it "training" doesn't get the point across.

In a few notable cases, he'd tell me to do something that I didn't want to do, or didn't think that I was even able to do. Despite my lack of intention to do it, he would point out later on that I had done it anyway, sometimes without noticing. He has shaped me in countless ways, so that when left to my own devices I naturally do things the way he wants me to. I don't even think of it as being obedient—it is just the way I *like* doing things, and it seems like I've always liked doing things this way.

At one point he officially told me that leaving him would be unthinkable. I already felt like I was so thoroughly bound to him that it wouldn't make any difference, but it was important to him. It wasn't just an order—like I said, it is brainwashing. For a year or so afterwards if I even speculated about hypothetically leaving I'd find myself thinking about laundry or singing a little song to myself. It became literally "unthinkable". I can think about leaving now, but I'm quite certain that if I tried to leave, I'd go mad fairly immediately. I realize that may be objectively true or it may not be, but I can't convince myself it isn't true any more than I can convince myself that putting my hand on the hot woodstove won't harm me.

Q: How does this internal enslavement thing work? What do you do?

Raven: First, this is a slow thing. It takes years. Be patient, know the slave really well, and keep up constant communication in order to be aware of every corner of their brain. You must remember that we're talking about conditioning here, whether hypnotic, repetitive, or whatever. Having seen it come on, I'd say that it doesn't happen like a switch flipping. It comes on slowly, and in the early stages a perceptive and self-aware submissive can watch it happening, and call it to the dominant's attention. That's what happened to us—Joshua noticed that he was becoming less and less able to disobey my orders and wishes, and pointed it out. It was a crossroads moment: did we want to go forward with this, or did we want to back up? There were things that I could have done to push it either way. If he'd wanted to make the choice himself, there were things that he could have done as well. We discussed the pros and cons, and decided to forge ahead into no-man's-land.

Once it's done, the mental conditioning is like a chain far stronger than anything physical. The mind is an amazing tool—just ask a hypnotist. It can convince us of all sorts of things that aren't objectively true, until they become so true for us that, for all practical purposes, they might as well be. Being a mentally conditioned slave in this way doesn't mean that you won't be unhappy or dissatisfied or dislike the way that your owner is doing things or think that they're a rotten owner or even hate them—consciously, anyway. You can run through all of those feelings in five minutes on a bad day, and if the conditioning is done right, you will still jump when they say so, even if you're hating them and yourself for doing it at the moment.

As it's a process in, so it's a process out. It can slowly lapse if the owner doesn't ever exercise their authority for a very long time, even subtly. It can be negatively affected by chemical mental illness, although how and to what extent may be variable.

I don't think that all the fetishy "slavey" activities actually do the work of the conditioning. I think that they exist to keep the submissive's attention long enough for the dominant to do the subtle work, which takes a long time and a lot of small moves. If the submissive isn't getting what they want out of the relationship while they can still leave, they'll do so.

This probably all sounds really cold and unromantic of me, and perhaps it is a very cold analysis of a process that was, in our case, done with a lot of care and consideration and love. But it didn't have to be that way; it could have been done without that and it still would have worked. "Worked" in the sense that he would still be owned—but then, you're both stuck with the situation (assuming that the dominant has any ethics at all), so it's best to think ahead to what you want before you both commit to it.

Another thing to remember is that if the submissive is actually in love with the dominant, well, love can feel a lot like enslavement when those brain drugs kick in. (Duh, all the song lyrics will tell you that.) The difference is that when those brain drugs die away, you're suddenly not so bound to them, whereas with internal enslavement it works no matter what you feel. That's what I ask people when they wonder if they're really internally enslaved: Do you love them? Imagine that you didn't. In fact, imagine that you hate them, and they're giving you an order that you really despise. What are you going to do, and how will you feel? Can you imagine yourself automatically obeying under those circumstances? If you can't imagine this, perhaps it's better that you not consider the issue until some of the love drugs have burned off (which takes about two years, according to the scientists).

In even the most vanilla and compatible of relationships, there will eventually come the day when (if only for an hour) you want nothing more than to punch your beloved in the face, repeatedly. (Or run away screaming, or poison their soup, or your version of that reaction.) It's normal, we're humans. That's the day when the owner should yank the chain, hard, and see if it holds. That's when you know who's really enslaved.

Q: What are some of the methods that you use?

Raven: Positive reinforcement for getting it right. No reinforcement for not getting it right. Lots of communication. A certain amount of hypnosis, and (for us) a small amount of magical binding. Getting him in the right receptive frame of mind, and telling him things in the right tone of voice, on a regular basis.

One of the most important things to remember is to have consistency in big messages. Little stuff can be inconsistent, but the big messages—you are mine, you can't leave, you must obey everything I say, you must be open to me in all things, you can trust me, I will let you know clearly when your behavior needs correction, I will keep you safe, I will make good judgments about your life, I am competent and able to handle this responsibility, etc.—must be very consistent. That means not doing things that undermine the messages, which means keeping a very close eye on the integrity of your own actions as the owner.

Getting the slave in a suggestible space on a regular basis and implanting information in them is one of my best tools. What "a suggestible space" means for each person is different, and must be discovered by the dominant. This requires a good deal of subtlety. I did a lot of work above-board, saying to Joshua, "OK, I'm going to put you into a mild trance state now and tell you X, which we've both decided is something that is good for you to totally internalize." However, sometimes I hit resistance. Then I'd have to do it subtly, without warning him. (This requires a huge amount of close observation of the slave, obviously.)

I'm more likely to be subtle in the way that I work with him, now that the major changes and made and we're down to little tweaks. The subtle approach is a lot more useful to me, but it does take a lot of work and strategy and observation. Also, because it makes Joshua feel like he's doing all this because it's naturally the way things ought to be done, sometimes he feels like I'm not controlling him very much at all, compared to some slaves whose writings he reads. He says this while automatically following a heavily boundaried and Raven-centered life that would horrify a free person.

The slave can actively help the process, or actively hinder it. As I've said earlier, they need to be heavily invested in giving their owner enough successes in changing them that the owner can figure out what works best for them. The more self-aware they are, the more they can give honest assessment as to what worked and how it worked. The more brutally honest they are about their motivations—especially the unflattering ones—the easier job their owner will have to change them. They need to be able to come up with good information on what it would take to become the sort of person who could do their job better.

So I'd say that just as the best quality they can have is adaptability, the best tool they can offer is deep self-awareness. The less self-aware they are, the harder they make it for their owner. Handing them the owner's manual, if only one chapter at a time, is a lot more helpful than hiding it, forgetting where you hid it, pretending you never had it, and handing them an attractive and flattering fake instead.

Joshua: My master will sometimes grab me in a certain way and tell me something in "Command Voice", and that generally works sort of like a hypnotic suggestion. That is, I find myself obeying it without intending to or even being all that aware that I am obeying it, even if I've forgotten he said it or at the time I didn't think it was going to work. He doesn't do this very often though. His training is more subtle than that.

My master is more likely to use touch to reinforce training than talk. His most common way of reinforcing me as *his*, with no boundaries, is by randomly grabbing my face and messing with it in a somewhat affectionate way, or absentmindedly fiddling with my body or clothing or hair. It isn't a directly sexual thing. It is the same attitude as when he picks up our cute little baby lambs and fondles them somewhat carelessly, without a whole lot of regard for whether the lamb is interested in it. There is a strong sense of "thing-ness" to it. It is deeply objectifying, but in a way that I find very comforting and right.

Later in this book, my master describes the internal training a slave as being like shaping one of those little bonsai trees—a long and subtle process, and the desired result is a form that looks entirely natural. The method desired by many slaves (myself included) is more of a Martha Stewart parody of bonsai, whacking all the limbs off a little tree and gluing them in an artful and uniform arrangement to a sturdy dowel—a quick but soulless creation which isn't sustainable. We want to be perfect slaves *now*, and that doesn't just happen. Some of the training methods out there will allow a slave to come to external obedience, but it doesn't stick around without constant external reinforcement.

My master uses a technique with me that he sometimes calls the Jedi Mind Trick or "programming", but brainwashing is just as good a term for it. It is a very natural and subtle process for us, though it used to be more explicit. In the earliest form, he would quickly put me into a light altered state and say something with a great deal of force of will behind it. We talked about the process at length, and I was an enthusiastic participant. I very much want to be the person he wants me to be. Struggling against my natural inclination is much harder than simply having his will laid on me, and works more reliably. It is very different than just wanting to obey and please him (which I do), or setting aside my own wants and preferences (which I do). I frequently act on my own preferences … but more and more of those preferences are things he's shaped. It gives the illusion of free will and many of the perks of free will, without sacrificing absolute obedience.

For instance, I am a little bummed right now because at his prompting I've enrolled in a class next term that conflicts with my community choir rehearsal. I never used to like singing before he forcibly enrolled me in the church choir where he sings. He'd deliberately altered me to enjoy singing, and I practically begged him to let me join this community choir. (It is hilarious when I step back to look at it.) My motivation in joining the community choir was not about pleasing him. While he loves music, he thinks this community choir is the height of dorky and has indicated that he is only humoring me in this. I joined because I now love singing and I genuinely want to improve at it. He's done this sort of thing to me countless times, and I expect I only notice a small portion of them. I don't think he's done much of the direct force-of-will thing with my sexual preferences because that is tricky and has had unfortunate side effects in the past. For that he does more gradual conditioning. Direct programming is the sort of thing where if you push too hard or don't think things through, you just make the person crazy.

One reason why he does this sort of training is that he prefers that I don't act "slavey" outside of sexplay or BDSM spaces. I am to basically act publicly like a vanilla lover who just so happens to see things his way, share his priorities and preferences, and enthusiastically do whatever he wants. I'm a slave that acts like a lover, rather than a lover that acts like a slave. The subtle conditioning and mental control is key to making this work seamlessly.

One point for experimenting dominants to remember: Subconscious messages are tricky, because sometimes negatives don't register correctly and less emotionally laden words get filtered out, so something like "You are not a loser" becomes "blah blah blah loser". Also, the subconscious is very able to hold mutually contradictory messages at the same time, so canceling out old patterns is harder than instilling new ones.

Q: Oh, come on. How do you know that you're not just fooling yourself about not being able to disobey?

Joshua: In the 99% of times when things are going well, there isn't a real noticeable difference because you genuinely want to obey, even if it isn't pleasant. The places where you notice it are the times when you don't want to obey. We've all got different boundaries about how defiant we can be, but the boundaries are there.

It isn't a matter of saying, "Oh, I could never disobey like that because I am a real slave." It is that once you get internally enslaved, when your master lays down a firm line, you are going to have extremely limited success in trying to cross it. Saying you have "no choice" is maybe misleading in this way. I think most IE slaves *can* "choose" to disobey, in that they can decide to disobey, but it is rare that they have much noticeable success in actually doing it. Either they find themselves obeying despite their intentions, or they have such a strong physical or emotional reaction that actually implementing the disobedient plan is almost impossible. I've seen the same types of reactions in so many IE slaves that I believe there is some sort of real mental shift that happens. Commonly reported reactions to attempted disobedience seem to be hyperventilating, nausea, vomiting, choking, passing out, headaches, disorientation, forgetfulness, feelings of tightness around the chest or neck, inability to breathe or speak or move.

Time for another example. I was professionally hypnotized a few months back, and I found the mental processes while under hypnosis are strangely similar to enslavement. At one point I was lying on the bed, the hypnotist told me I couldn't move my legs, and I thought, "Okay, I'll play along. It'd be pretty rude to move my legs when she's trying to help me out." Then she told me to try to move my legs. I struggled with whether I should really try or keep playing along, and with great difficulty I decided that if I wanted to I *could* move my legs. In fact, I put all my force of will behind it and successfully wiggled my right toes an almost imperceptible amount. (At least, I believe that I did. No one else saw it and I didn't have my glasses on so I can't be sure.) My internal reaction at the time was, "See! It didn't work! I moved my toes!" When I mentioned this afterwards the hypnotist pointed out what a tiny percentage of my normal range of motion this was, and asked if I thought I could have got up and walked away. Nope. Honestly, if I had wanted to get away, I would have tried rolling myself off the bed before it ever would have occurred to me to stand up.

For me, this is very much what it is like trying to directly disobey when you are internally enslaved.

Q: If your master decided to change something about you that you didn't want to be changed, wouldn't it still be your choice to some extent to comply with it?

Joshua: If my master decided to change something like this, it would not be done suddenly. It would be a subtle art of reinforcement and shaping. Because he prefers to get my input on these things, he'd let me know that he intended to do it, and if I had no objections he'd drop the subject. If I had objections, we'd talk about them, and he would take them into account when making his decision. (That wouldn't make it my choice; it is his choice to pay attention to my opinions or not.) I wouldn't be aware he was changing anything until long afterwards. If someone pointed it out, I might be able to notice that I am different than what I once was, but it wouldn't feel like something externally imposed. It'd feel like a natural progression, or a change I made in myself because it felt more natural to be this way.

I know this because he's already done it to me. Now I have a sort of cheerfully lazy acceptance of it. It is an unpleasant lot of work for me to obey when it goes against my natural inclination. I'll do it because I am obedient, but by definition I don't like doing things I don't like doing! On the other hand, it is no work at all for me to let my natural inclination be passively changed. Then I do it "of my own free will" as it were, and everyone is happy.

Q: What if you order the slave to do something that they find terribly repugnant? Could they disobey if the psychological stress was extreme enough? Would the order break the enslavement? If it won't, what would?

Raven: If Joshua did not do what I ordered, it would be because he *couldn't*, not because he chose not to. Knowing that, I would not ask him to do something that he felt was ethically wrong, unless I felt that it was an absolute emergency—and in all the time we've been together, nothing has been *that* much of an emergency! Frankly, my moral code is stricter than his. Well, than his was before he got himself owned. Now my code is by default his code.

If I asked him to do something and he said, "Please, sir, don't make me do that, I don't think it's right," I would let him explain to me why he thought it was wrong. (We will go under the assumption here that I disagree and think it's right.) I then have two options: convince him that it is right, or make him do it anyway. I would go for #1 first. If it didn't work I'd say never mind. Not worth the mess I'd have to clean up afterwards from him feeling awful because he did something he considered that bad. Would I attempt to condition him into changing his mind about an ethical issue? No, because that's sleazy. To do that would be a sign of someone who shouldn't be in charge of another human being.

Whether a slave can disobey if the situation is bad enough ... I don't know whether I can make that absolute definition for the entirety of consensual slavehood, or even all of the internally enslaved. People are too different. One might assume that if a slave got to that point, then their owner's hold on them was definitely cracking, if not entirely cracked. But I can speak for myself: If my slave deliberately disobeyed me, it would say to me that they were no longer internally enslaved by me. Even if I had held their will, I'd now lost it, and I no longer owned them. That would mean backing up and starting from scratch and renegotiating things, for me anyway.

But there are things that can break internal enslavement. One is a complete undermining of the trust involved that led the submissive to make the deal in the first place. As IE is a long, slow process, the losing of trust is also usually not a one-shot deal. If the heretofore trustworthy owner does one bad thing, it won't generally make the slave internally unenslaved. It will make them upset and terrified and still bound, a pretty awful place to be in. If it goes on with multiple betrayals over time, the trust, and thus the enslavement, will be worn away and they will be able to leave. (And probably should!) The other thing that wears away enslavement is the owner not bothering to keep up with the work of it. If the owner quits reinforcing (often because they get lazy) it slowly wears off. In this case, you'll sometimes see a slave start to rebel, partly because their independent survival instincts are reasserting themselves, partly because they want to know where their limits are now, and partly as a plea to the owner to keep up their end of the bargain.

Q: Is this about "breaking" your slave?

Raven: You mean like "breaking" a horse? While there is a lot of debate over the definition of that word, let me say that "breaking" usually assumes that the individual is traumatized until they can no longer disobey. This is not *at all* what I've done. My slave is not "broken" at all; he's *changed.* Formed. Sculpted. Remolded. All done over a long period of time, tiny bit by tiny bit. No breakage necessary. I've altered his will subtly, over time, with conditioning. I've also altered his desires and preferences to be more like mine. That doesn't mean turning the slave into a pile of Jello. I assure you that if anyone tried to force Joshua to do something that was against his ethics, or self-destructive, you wouldn't get very far at all. His will is still there when it comes to other people, and most other situations. It's only been specifically altered in these few instances.

Really, the bonsai tree metaphor that is the title of this chapter is quite apt. You set context and limits, and then you encourage them to grow. And if you've set the limits right (and you keep delicately, subtly adjusting them all the time), and you've encouraged growth right, you get the tree you want, happy and healthy. Of course, in order to be a work of art, it had to be radically pruned, and this does mean that it wouldn't work so well to stick it back into the wild without a period of adaptation. But that's the price you pay for a beautiful thing to keep in your house.

The problem is when you try to do it to a specimen that isn't right for bonsai, or you try to make a pine into a willow.

The other problem is that this is way too much work for most dominants.

Q: Is being internally enslaved better or more serious or "hardcore" than a relationship where the slave chooses again every day to continue? How different are the two states for practical purposes?

Joshua: I have a fairly strict definition of what an owned slave is, and I find it useful to have space with people who share that definition to discuss practical and psychological aspects of ownership. People in non-ownership based D/s relationships have different struggles and issues. There is an area of overlap, and I can usefully discuss life in service with someone whether they are owned or not, but there are things that just don't translate.

See, I always considered voluntary honor-bound service to be more prestigious than "slavery", and I resisted the label of slave for quite some time. I felt the implication that I might have to be held by force to be an insult to my loyalty and commitment. Then I became a slave, and here I am. I'm not sure if I still consider voluntary ongoing submission to be more prestigious. It is what it is. I think one can achieve a higher ideal of pure service through active submission, because few masters really give as much of a damn about pure service in and of itself. They are generally more practical than that. Being a slave is easier, in a way. A voluntary submissive needs to be a stronger, more dedicated person to achieve excellence in their role. A slave need only be malleable.

I don't know if this will make any sense, but I'll try to use this metaphor. To me it is like the difference between being a soldier and a monk. A soldier will be pushed through his reluctance and wavering, by force if needed. A lesser man can become a fine soldier. It is easier to be a bad monk, so you have to be a better man to be a good monk. Some monastic orders are stricter than others and some will push you harder than others, but no one is going to force you to do anything at gunpoint. You need to maintain your own dedication.

Is one of them better than the other? No. They are just different. But if the soldier and the monk talk about their struggles with dedication and loyalty, they are going to come to some misunderstandings and confusion if one of them insists he is just the same as the other.

In some ways I still feel like it is more honorable and praise-worthy to serve someone entirely of your own free will. This kind of mind control seems too easy, from the submissive point of view. Most of the time I feel like I can do whatever I like - it just never occurs to me to do the things I've been ordered not to do.

I do have a fair amount of willpower, and that is of great use in my daily life, but it is totally irrelevant in my obedience to him. I'd get along just as well without it. So if one is to think of "obedience" as a virtue that a person cultivates, I can tell you from personal experience that without free will it becomes a meaningless concept. To try a different metaphor, this would be like saying a fish is obedient for staying in its fishbowl. No. A dog who stays in an unfenced yard is obedient. The fish is just content to be in a bowl. I think that for submissives who no longer need to give ongoing voluntary consent, the virtue to cultivate is contentment.

Raven: Can I say again (and again, and again!) that this is not for everyone, or even for most D/s people? Can I say again that no one needs to feel that they are "less" in any way because they do not practice IE, or because they (as a submissive) want to keep open that last door of being able to get out if necessary? For the vast majority of people, that's the right thing to do. Don't let anyone tell you that it isn't, and don't assume that message is there when it isn't. There are many different and equally valid ways to do a power dynamic. People should do what is healthiest for them. There, have I said it enough? Every submissive who has been reading this section and feeling insecure because their preferred level of power dynamic is less absolute should now roll up a newspaper and beat themselves with it for being silly.

I know that one of the dangers in Joshua and myself writing about IE techniques is that some people will use this information to prove how much more hardcore they are than other people, and that yet others will assume that people are doing that even when they aren't. I'd like to take a newspaper to all of them, too.

Q: Do you keep your slave locked up? Does he ever get to leave the house and do normal things?

Raven: Because he has no more freedom, I am paradoxically able to allow him a whole lot of "freedom". He leaves most days to go to school (getting the degrees and certifications that I want him to get, so as to better serve me), or work (earning money that I can spend as I choose but he can't touch without permission), or shopping (to buy what he knows I want), or errands (to help me with my work), or to drive me places. Because of my increasing joint pain, I can't drive long distances, and we live on the edge of nowhere, so he is my chauffeur. The car is in my name, but he's the one who drives and maintains it.

To some people, this would look like he's an ordinary person living an ordinary life. It's not. Every single thing he does is bounded by my wishes and expectations. Every place he goes, I chose and ordered him to go there. Every moment that he works or studies, all his effort goes into making sure that he is enacting my orders to the best of his ability. The real truth kicks in here: He can't decide *not* to do any of those things. A free person can drop out of school, quit a job, decide to skip that trip to the post office and go home. He can't.

He handles the money, too, because he's good at details and because I have better things to do. This means that he has a list of bills to pay, and he does it. He gets no allowance of his own. If he wants to buy something, he lets me know and I decide if it gets bought. For me it's rather like being a medieval samurai who didn't want to lower himself to bother with money; his wife handled all of that. I just periodically ask him about the state of the superfluous funds and he tells me. I decide where it goes; he is my instrument in doing that. I'm the brain and he is the hands. It's that simple and smooth. We are a good team.

There is a collar around his neck, although you'll never see it. It's invisible, and it tightens around his throat every time he even thinks about making a move that I wouldn't approve of. There are chains on his body, equally invisible, that physically stop him in his tracks in the same situations. I don't need to put anything made of metal on him. My invisible chains are better. And since I don't give a damn what other people think of how "real" our M/s is, it doesn't matter if they're all invisible. Like the invisible fence for the dog, eventually they internalize the boundary until they'd stay in the yard even if you forgot to put the collar on them.

So, while I can't speak for anyone else, I know that I trust Joshua with more freedoms because he is so absolutely enslaved. To me, there's a lot of power in knowing that someone can be sent out into the mundane world, with almost no reminders of their slavery in place—no collar, no chains, no fetishy gear, no locked door, no master anywhere in sight—and they'll be just as enslaved and unable to do anything but follow their orders exactly as they were told. That's power. It's like the saying that I love: To have is riches, to be able to do without is power. It's *easy* to feel slavish when you're surrounded by the trappings. It's much harder without any of them (well, all right, he has a tattoo on his arm with my name on it) and thus reifies how strong my power really is.

This isn't to say, of course, that there's something wrong with trappings. If they are fulfilling for you, heap them on with my blessings. Naked, unadorned power just happens to be my own personal fetish.

Q: Do you always have to tell the truth to your master?

Joshua: Yes, because that's what he's ordered, and I can't disobey. However, the way in which that command works on a daily basis is quirky and amusing. I've developed a crazy level of literal, unbiased honesty. Even when I say perfectly true things, if I slant them in a way that is more favorable to me or if I present information in a leading manner, I get an uneasy feeling. It doesn't seem to matter that my master doesn't give a damn about the tiny inaccuracy or possibly misleading phrasing. It is just part of the enslavement process.

I've found that I can figure out if I'm lying to myself by looking my master in the eye and telling him whatever it is that I'm hoping is true. Even when I feel like I really believe it is true, if deep down some part of me knows it isn't, I can barely get the words out. If I really look him in the eye and tell him something like "So-and-so wouldn't mind if I borrowed her..." and my heart starts racing like crazy before I can finish the sentence, then I know I don't really believe it.

It means that the internal enslavement orders are self-monitoring. For example, there's the issue of motivation. My master doesn't much care if I do chores and things with the purest motivation. I can grumble all I like so long as I'm doing the job while I grumble. But when I'm grumbling, I'm very aware that I am doing something wrong. He doesn't mind it, but it is corrosive to me. The more I do it, the worse it gets. It weighs on my conscience, and I have to stop.

Q: How do you approach disagreements and conflicts in such a relationship?

Joshua: I've found that when I disagree with the way I have been told to do something, it is because I have different priorities than my master. Over time I have internalized more and more of his priorities, but it is useful to me to understand why his decisions made sense from that standpoint if I haven't yet internalized the particular priorities that are a problem. From there, obedience comes naturally and gracefully.

I know that some masters do not care to share their motivations or reasons with their slaves, but mine has always done so quite readily, time permitting. Also, a mindful servant can pick up on patterns of behavior even when the master doesn't care to explain every last thing. While I am expected to obey whether I agree with my master or not, he has a strong preference for me agreeing with him and believing him to be right. He doesn't think highly of a person who would gladly serve someone they continually believe to be in error. That means that I am allowed to discuss things, and even argue, so long as it stays respectful. In the end, it's his say, but I agreed to that in the beginning, so I knew what I was getting into. But we do a lot of processing.

In some service situations it is best to develop a habit of instinctive, unquestioning obedience. In others, a certain inquisitiveness is more appropriate. I find the second to be useful in developing a deep enslavement dynamic. One works from the outside in—you first create the appearance of obedience, supported by external motivation, and this is meant to bring about the internal desire to obey and act rightly. The other works from the inside, attempting to give the innate desire to obey a natural mode of expression, which is intended to bring about a strong internally-motivated obedience. Rather than suppressing the will of the slave, you align it with the master's will.

Coming to a deep state of obedience is a slow process by any method! I found that an embarrassing amount of my drive to be perfect, to be the "slaviest" slave, the best boy ever, was motivated by vanity and pride, not a pure desire to serve. That has had to be pruned away. A genuine desire to serve has a great degree of humility to it, and patience.

Q: Does the internal enslavement process change the slave's core self, or just the exterior?

Joshua: Oh boy. My master asked me to respond to this one, but it is really complicated for me to make a sensible answer.

During the two years when I met my master, there was so much change in my life—ways in which I changed, and ways in which my circumstances changed me. Some of them are clearly due to my master, and some predate meeting him, but it all happened at around the same time. A year prior to meeting my master, I was a loud-mouthed, gender-deviant punk with a bright orange mohawk, offensive slogans written on my clothes, a big nose ring and plugs in my ears. I was in school for computer engineering, worked in that field, and supported my boyfriend who I insisted do 90% of the housework for me. I had been into the leather scene since my teens, generally up for whatever crazy play was going on that weekend. I considered my relationship with my first master, in my mid-teens, to be my lesson in why I was not suited to (or interested in) heavy D/s. I just liked kinky sex.

A year later, I had moved from the city to a little farmhouse many states away, happily pledging to spend the rest of my life in service. I grew my hair out in its natural color, removed all visible piercings, and started dressing in simple, wholesome clothing. I became sincerely, devoutly and passionately religious, which boggled my entire family. I had a falling out with them which took years to resolve to the point where most of them will speak civilly to me. I legally changed my full name to something entirely different than the one I was given at birth ... and those are only the changes that I feel like discussing in public.

I was relatively young during all this, and while I'd been living on my own for some time, in many ways I came to full adulthood under my master's ownership. That confuses the issue, but perhaps in a good way. It meant that most people attributed most of the changes to me growing up, rather than me losing my mind or joining a cult. If I had been in my thirties, I think more people would have worried. Of course, I moved many states away during all this, and aside from my family (who I rarely see) there is only one friend who has really known me on both sides of that transition.

So ... did this change my core self? That's hard to say. My ideas about who I was at my core changed substantially, but not entirely. There are foundations of my personality that are the same. But there are also things that I could have sworn were foundational that just aren't there anymore. There isn't even a hole where they were. It is possible that I was wrong about who I really was—young people often are—but I think that some deep things did change. I don't feel like the person I am now is who I was all along, buried under layers of "not me" until my master uncovered the "real me". Maybe for other slaves that is true, but I've never felt that way.

There is certainly a strong feeling of continuity between who I was then and who I am now, but I do remember one evening some years ago when I looked at myself in the mirror and had a little "Who am I? What the hell happened to me?" meltdown. It wasn't that I disliked the changes—I was happier than I'd ever been in my life—but I hadn't noticed that much changing going on. It hit me all at once that night, and I think I was more scared about the not-noticing than about the changing. But the panic passed by morning, and even though I've changed much more since that night, I haven't felt that way again. It taught me that who I am is malleable. I've learned not to identify too strongly with the superficial markers of who I am, and pay more attention to whether who I am now is good and right for where I am now, rather than whether it is the "real me" or the same as it was last year or the year before.

Q: So you've talked a lot about using subtle rather than direct forms of control. How does this work for the slave in the equation? Which do they prefer? Which works better for extracting obedience?

Raven: Joshua likes overt control, because it gives him psychological satisfaction while it's happening. I still use a certain amount of overt control for short-term things, but for long-term changes I prefer to be subtler, because it works. Overt control doesn't always last past the controlling period, and it has a much higher level of creating resistance.

To be fair, a different type of slave might do better with more direct methods, especially if the need for perceived control is very high. If the owner wants to use subtle methods in that case, they might think about having strong, obvious, direct control in a number of less important areas, and meanwhile work on subtle control of larger and deeper ones. It could be seen almost like a diversion, keeping the slave focused elsewhere while the more delicate work is done.

Actually, he sometimes does miss the overt control ... sometimes to the point of entirely forgetting that control is even there. Joshua was once reading over my shoulder while I wrote an email about how boundaried and controlled his life is with all my rules, and said to me, "I think you're overstating the case a little."

Me: But isn't every one of these rules true? Not to mention all the ones I didn't put in?

Him: Well, yeah.

Me: Could you decide to disobey any of them?

Him: Well, no. But it's not a big deal. It's not like I want to disobey them. I mean, yeah, I can't cut my hair and I can't buy stuff without permission and I have the career you want me to have and I report in to you all the time and I can't have orgasms without you there, and I couldn't leave and all that, but it's not like it's a big deal.

Me: Hmmm. Josh, would anybody you know who is *not* a slave happily go along with all those rules and be fine with never being able to disobey them? Anyone? Would my wife?

Him: Well ... no. Oh.

We talked more, but it finally came down to the point that I alluded to. When you do it the subtle way, the slave often doesn't feel like they're being controlled. They settle into a routine that would make any free person scream and run, and feel like "it's not a big deal, so I don't feel very controlled." So one lessens the struggle of resistance, but pays for it with less "control satisfaction" from the slave. Still, I'm happy with my methods. He isn't terribly upset over this supposed lack of being controlled (snort!) and if he gets upset about it, I'll see if I can fixate his need for it on something else. It really made me laugh, though. When it becomes natural, by whatever means, they just forget how far off "normal" it is.

Q: Could someone be internally enslaved in a long-distance relationship? Would you even call them a slave?

Joshua: I tend to call anyone who is actively in the enslavement process a "slave". Some are just further along in the process and some are better at their jobs, but until they demonstrate they are not enslaved, I'm happy to give them the courtesy of the title. (Whittling the pool of "real slaves" down further and further and further doesn't seem to benefit anyone.)

In any case, you don't really know how strong any power is until it is tested in some way. So you explore the limits of the situation, if only in honest discussion. If you've got a slave who is capable of very honest self-reflection, talk to them. Ask hard questions about how they'd feel about certain orders that are on or past the edge of their comfort zone. The hypothetical novice slave will usually give you a quick bright-eyed, "Of course, Sir! I will obey you in every way, Sir," but you can't take that seriously because they don't really know yet. A little further along and our hypothetical novice says "What? You wouldn't! Right? Please tell me you wouldn't ask that." At this point you know they are really understanding things but not quite there yet. Eventually our not-so-novice slave responds by getting real quiet and saying something like, "Holy crap ... I *would* do that if you asked, wouldn't I?" That shows they are in the process of coming to terms with their internal enslavement. Once they get through that they can give the "Of course, Ma'am," and really mean it.

My main problem with long-distance relationships is that the potential for unwitting self-deception (and intentional misrepresentation) is so high. It is very easy to maintain an illusion with someone who you rarely see. Long-distance masters will generally say they have complete control over their slaves and the slave would leave their spouse and quit their job and move to Ohio with them if they commanded it; they just don't want it. I'd wager that 90% of them are wrong and at least half of them know it. There can be good reasons for keeping things long-distance, but in most cases I think the reason is that the master doesn't want the responsibility of a full-time M/s relationship and/or doesn't actually have enough control to pull it off. (Temporary long-distance is a different thing. That is more a matter of planning and patience.)

Q: Joshua, do you think that you'll become even more submissive as time goes on?

Joshua: To me, being "more submissive" would mean being more able to set my will aside. An example of this was a slave who spoke eloquently about how "breaking" his will had changed his service. Before, if he was used "inefficiently"—first being summoned to fetch the domme's glasses, then a few minutes later being summoned to fetch her a sweater, then a few minutes later to make coffee for her—he was resentful. Afterwards, he simply felt honored to be summoned for any task.

This sort of thing is about being without will. "Breaking" is one way to get there, but it tends to leave you with a damaged person and the ethics of it are questionable, to say the least. For the process to be real and healthy, it must go slowly and mindfully.

Being without will, to whatever extent possible, is a very desirable state for me. When I feel particularly willful, I don't like it, since to be well-behaved while feeling willful is an unpleasant struggle. It feels so good to be able to serve my master wholly, and I know I am better able to serve him when I'm not fighting with my own ego. But from the beginning of our relationship, my master has said that he does not want me to go past a certain point of submission. I am required to retain a certain amount of will and individuality because he finds me more useful and interesting that way. That's a hard point for me to find sometimes. My natural set-point is currently a few marks higher than what I think my master would like, but not too far off. He can hold me at whatever point he likes if he's paying attention to me, but he tends to leave me to my own devices unless he requires absolute obedience on a given thing.

I'd like to think that I could go further down this road, and that it would feel even more natural to me than it does now.

Mind, Heart, and Spirit: Creating Depth

Values

Q: Are owners better than slaves? Do slaves really think that their owners are superior people? Aren't they human, just like everyone else? And as a corollary, should a dominant strive to be right more often, and a better person in general, than their slave?

Raven: When people say "better", the first question that pops into my head is "better at what?" Obviously anyone that I meet is likely to be better than me at something, if only rattling off Pokemon characters. But I would guess that what slaves mean when they refer to their owners as "better" is likely to be an arbitrary collection of qualities that have meaning only for them.

When I asked Joshua—some time ago, actually—whether he actually believed that I was a superior human being to him, he said yes, unequivocally yes. I was rather taken aback, actually. I've had it drummed into my head that all people are equal in general worthiness before the Powers That Be, etc. etc. But when I probed further, I found that he wasn't talking about any high impersonal scale, but a deeply personal one. I think that we need to make that distinction here.

He pointed out that I have a higher IQ, better self-control, better judgment in decisions, more experience with relationships, more strength of will, better ability to plan, greater ambition, more competence at handling people, better memory, fourteen years more experience, stricter ethics and honor, more creativity, more spiritual knowledge, and more of an ability to make an impact on the world, than him. To him, that says "better". Never mind that he is a computer geek and I am such a Luddite that I can barely figure out how to do my email; never mind that I find him smart, insightful, and eminently perceptive; never mind that I could never make homemade mayonnaise like his. To him, the above are the factors that make me "better" in his definition...

...and yes, he set that definition before he met me. He stated firmly that if I hadn't been better at him at most of those things—especially the judgment, willpower, and self-control—he would not have come into being my slave. He might have served me consensually, but he would not have felt that I was worthy of turning his entire life and being over to. In order to be worthy of service in his mind, his future master had to be better than him at these particular things, or he wouldn't—couldn't—be mastered by him.

Considering that if you end up a consensual-nonconsent-type slave, where the last big decision you will make is what sort of person to give yourself to ... why wouldn't you want to add your power to that of someone whom you felt was "better than you" at whatever collection of traits is important to your personal definition of worthiness? A submissive had better darn well have a definition of worthiness, whatever that may be, for their own safety. I strongly suggest that unattached subs make a thoughtful list of the traits that their ideal master should be superior at. That list will vary from sub to sub, and that's all right.

I am simply happy that the collection of traits that he needed a master to be "superior" in was one that I could cover. If he needed a master to be superior to him in things like height, or handsomeness, or computer ability, or wealth, or health, or physical condition, or organizational ability, or penis size, I'd be pretty well out of luck. Or, at least, he would be serving someone else and not me. (Someone tall and built and rich and well hung, maybe.) So it all depends on what the slave feels are the traits that make their owner "better" than them.

The flip side of that question is, indeed, whether the owner should strive to be better and more often right than the slave. I would never speak for other dominants, but for myself, in my own M/s relationship ... yes, I do hold myself to that. Otherwise, why the heck would an submissive want to do what I say and let me make all their life decisions for them? If my general life judgment about how things should go over the long term is worse than theirs (or at the least, no better), then why are they here and not with someone whose judgment is better than theirs?

Before all the dominants reading this decide to kill me, let me disclaimer again that this is only the way that I feel for myself, about my own situation. There may also be something to the fact that my M/s relationship, while it is filled with deep love on both sides, is not love-based. By that, I mean that it isn't love that sustains any part of the M/s. (The love sustains other things.) To be fair, some submissives have honestly answered the above rhetorical question with, "Because I love them, and it's more important to me to serve someone I love and who loves me than someone who is necessarily a better person than me." For them, the emotions were all-important. In contrast, I don't think that Joshua could bring himself to serve someone that he loved, but only loved and didn't respect as a superior. A submissive with a strong moral code who values morality over feelings would likely not allow themselves to be taken by a dominant without a code that was as strong or greater. So, again, it comes around to what the submissive values when they begin the process of giving themselves over.

Continually striving to be the worthy of this privilege doesn't mean that I have to have better specialized skills or knowledge than my slave in any practical arena. The areas where it is most important for me, personally, to be better than my slave are A) general life judgment and B) moral code of honor. Because that's where the navigation is, so to speak. All the rest is just delegatable. Perhaps it will make more sense to say that for myself, a moral screwup would be much worse than it would for my slave. He can afford to make the "usual" percentage of moral screwups; I don't feel that I can. I feel that my ratio of code-of-honor foulups has to be significantly less than the average, or even above-average person ... because more rides on my decisions, and I have more ability to do harm. In general, I would assume that a leader of people should be held to a higher code of honor than the average joe to whom no one listens. However, this becomes extra crucial when it's leading people who no longer have the free will to walk out when they feel like it.

Joshua: There's a very important distinction to be made here. Many folks have the idea that they ought to believe that all masters are inherently better than all slaves, and this is especially problematic if the only requirement for being a master is calling yourself one, whether you have a slave or not. I'm not sure how I'd feel about a M/s pair where both believed the slave was a better person by some mutually meaningful criteria, but I suppose that it's possible, and my discomfort with that is probably my own issues.

Some people have a strong emotional reaction to the idea that any one person might be any better than any other person (in an unqualified sense of "better than"). In our culture, the justification for humane treatment of individuals is based on the idea that all people are of equal worth. It's entirely possible, however, to believe in the importance of treating all people well while still believing that they might have differing value. (The problems come in when some people, or entire groups of people, are seen as having almost no value at all.) Beyond that, people in any situation of less power often like to find solace in the idea of their own unrecognized superiority. While this can be a sanity-saver in a nonconsensual situation, it's not appropriate for consensual M/s ... but it often leaks over anyway, out of habit. For some people, believing that someone else might be better than them in large, important ways would simply send them into a spiral of self-loathing.

The flip side to seeing some people as better than yourself is seeing yourself as better than some people. However, this doesn't mean that you can treat them badly. In fact, part of your position as their superior is based on how well you treat them. That's part of noblesse oblige. I don't so much see it as a class hierarchy across D/s, though. That is, I don't see dominants as superior to submissives in general, and I don't feel that dominants are automatically owed any greater respect or deference than submissives. I suspect I could adapt quite readily to habitual deference to my social "betters", but not when the alleged "betters" are entirely self-appointed and largely without responsibilities, qualifications or meaningful claim to authority beyond that of the average person.

Personally? Yes, I believe that my master is a better person than me. I also believe that his intrinsic worth is a substantial amount higher than mine, and that he is more important to the world than I am. He isn't better than me at everything, but he is better in the ways that count. (It's another one of those areas where we differ; he's a little uncomfortable with the fact that I see him this way.) This isn't something that troubles me or makes me feel bad about myself. If I considered him my peer, I suspect I would resent his control over me on some level.

I was recently reading a book on Victorian-era domestic service, and one servant of the time had commented that the reason service wasn't degrading was that you were serving your betters. The writer said that a person cannot be happy continually deferring to the will of an equal, and that the knowledge that the master is in some sense greater than the servant is what makes their service an honorable and worthwhile thing. The writer said that being ordered about by an equal (or someone you are superior to) and being expected to defer to them in all things would be degrading and insulting. Speaking of lady's maids, a paper of the time commented that "one woman cannot happily do the will of another woman simply because it is her will without looking up to her to some degree."

That may not be true for everyone (and probably isn't true for most), but it is true for me. (Perhaps I'm just awfully Victorian in my internal views. I certainly ended up dressing the part, at any rate.) I don't consider myself my master's equal. I consider his goals and desires to be more important than mine. I believe he rightly holds authority over me for reasons that go beyond his assertion of being dominant, and that no good whatsoever could come of our situations being reversed. However, that doesn't make me feel bad about myself. My self-esteem is fine. I'm a good and valued servant, after all; my master's prize possession. I can see that for a sub whose self-esteem was triggered by being seen as socially inferior, they'd have to believe differently out of self-defense.

I've found that the "bigger" a decision is, the bigger the difference between us in judgment. In utterly trivial decisions, I tend to have superior judgment, because I pay closer attention to those things and put more thought into them. In fairly important decisions, he's right a good deal more often than I am, though we often both can come up with a workable solution.

In major decisions, not only is he right vastly more often that I am, when he is wrong, he is far less wrong than I am. That is, his failures in judgment don't end up all that badly, because he's made contingency plans and whatnot. Mine have the potential to go terribly badly, and have. To me, this is the one area where a dominant absolutely must be skillful, because the long-term goals are their job. Figuring out where the lives of the two people involved are going to go, and how to get them there, is the single biggest responsibility they have. A dominant who can't do that well is a disaster waiting to happen.

Q: What about objectifying a slave? Isn't that degrading? Slaves are human beings, not inanimate objects.

Raven: When people object to objectification, it seems like they are having a hard time with the idea of a slave as "property"... and all that comes with that, including the idea that property might have different levels of value, especially to different people.

One of the problems that I have with most discussions of objectifying people is that these discussions never seem to take into account the incredibly variable and utterly irrational attitude that human beings have toward actual inanimate possessions. Most of these discussions treat the matter as if the person was automatically to be valued about as much as a crumpled Dixie cup.

But humans have had far different attitudes toward nonhuman property. The first letter in the Germanic runic alphabet (which is basically the Indo-European cultural map), Fehu, means movable property (not land). It is shaped like cows' horns, and is a glyph for cattle. From earliest times, our stuff has come first.

There are inanimate objects that people worship as sacred and kiss in reverence. There are objects that people kill others to take, or would kill if someone tried to take them. There are objects that have huge body counts, and are considered more valuable than all the lives sacrificed to gain them. There are objects of sentimental value that people would grab first in a house fire, before their pets or perhaps even other people. There are objects that people go without luxuries or even staples in order to afford. There are objects that people obsess over to the exclusion of interacting with other humans. A teenager who kills another teen for his running shoes certainly sees those shoes as having more importance, more individuality, and more worth than the guy wearing them.

We like to pretend that our values fall into a nice clean hierarchy, with people at the top, then animals (perhaps in descending order depending on physical complexity and intelligence), and then inanimate objects—but it isn't true. Not in the least. If we saw all, or even most, objects as interchangeable or of equal worth, we could all happily live in communes where they share all belongings, and no commercial could ever convince anyone to buy anything.

We don't see even types of objects as interchangeable. If I tell you that all cars are interchangeable, so I'm going to take yours and you can have mine, you will probably object strenuously. Every item we see, we judge on an inner (and very irrational) scale. Some of those objects, for some of us, will rank higher than some people. Period.

So to be realistic, and actually face the (ugly?) truth, treating a person like an object is as good or bad as treating them like a person. At least, that's how we really see things, when we're honest. Many things are set as more valuable than many people. The hierarchy is much more muddled than we like to believe.

So ... what it's really about is ... what sort of object do I treat my slave like? If I treat my slave like a believing Catholic treats a holy relic, is that the kind of objectification that most people would have in mind? Do I treat them like an expensive car that I dreamed of owning for two decades? An old junker that will likely fall apart at any moment? A half-million-dollar diamond necklace? A piece of plastic Tupperware? The family Bible that was passed down through twenty generations? A piece of expensive but hard-working machinery, bought for its reliability and multiple uses? The rag doll that your beloved mother made for you just before she passed away from a terrible disease? Your computer with the endlessly fascinating collection of video games? Your good-luck rabbit's foot? A crumpled Dixie cup? This is all without bringing in the even more difficult issue of animism—the idea that some inanimate objects have indwelling souls, which puts a whole 'nother slant on possessions.

My point is ... it's never all that simple, because possessions, and one's attitude toward them, will always be rather irrational, personal, and eccentrically individual. So the concept of objectification is a lot more complicated than we like to think.

Love

Q: Should owners love their slaves? Isn't it better to love them than not to love them?

Raven: I've had submissives that I loved and ones I didn't love. Currently I love my boy very passionately. I didn't expect to, although I hoped it would happen. I was his first experience of falling in love; he had expected a non-emotional service relationship, and was guarded enough that he would probably have been able to pull it off ... but Aphrodite had other ideas.

If I acquired other slaves, I would not want a deep romantic love-relationship with them at this time. On the other hand, I would still have their best interests at heart. It isn't love that makes me do good in relationships. I am perfectly capable of loving someone and hurting them terribly out of selfishness ... and so are many other people. It's my honor that keeps a slave safe with me, and unlike love which may wax and wane, my honor is always there like a leash. So I know from experience that I can have a submissive and not be in love with them, and still treat them very well. It would all have to be worked out beforehand, of course. I've had sub/servants before with this arrangement, just not property.

If property fell in love with me and I didn't return the feeling, how would I react? Well, it would depend on how they handled it. If they handled it sensibly, then it would be fine. If they couldn't stop hoping that I would ever change, and they let those dreams make them do dumb things ... then I would have to let them go, and tell them to go find someone who would be in love with them, since that was clearly what they needed.

I'd like to point out that in much of the gay male leather community, the idea that D/s or M/s ought to be, or is usually, accompanied by love is ludicrous. That's an entire demographic of people, many of whom are in relationships that I would consider deep M/s, for whom love might or might not happen. (Heterosexual female submissives, on the other hand, are usually the ones who can't imagine submission without love and romance as well.) If you ask submissive gay men why they are in a relationship with M/s but no love, they may give you different answers. Some will say that it turns them on. Some will say that the control is important enough for them that love is not as important. Some will say that service is the most important thing. I also know some gay male leather daddies who take women—straight and lesbian—into service for them, and they have neither sexual nor love relationships with them. It's pure service.

For the positional service-oriented subs, it's not unusual for love to be secondary. Joshua is like that. The fact that we are in love with each other was at first very disconcerting to him; he didn't want it and was afraid it would interfere. It's now comfortable for him, but still secondary. In public places where people would not understand our relationship, he'd really rather refer to me as his employer than as his lover. I feel differently, so it goes differently, but I'm aware that would be his preference.

I have read the theories of the no-love school of M/s—the idea that if the master and slave fall in love, the love may render the master too soft-hearted to be completely firm with the slave. While I can understand and even agree that this is an issue, those folks have little advice for whom masters and slaves are supposed to fall in love with (I actually get the idea from their writing that masters are supposed to be too tough to fall in love with anyone), or what to do if you're the sort of person for whom deep love and connection is bound up with very strong levels of possessiveness and the requirement of complete vulnerability of the partner—in other words, people who can only fully love a slave. I expect that they, too, would find me emotionally "wrong". Ah well.

Joshua: Weighing in on the love issue: One of my master's hopes before accepting me fully into intimate service was that I would fall deeply in love with him. He didn't tell me this at the time, because he thought it would put inappropriate pressure on me. He only told me later, when I was lamenting that (in my opinion) our emotional entanglement got in the way of "pure service". He loves all the things he truly owns, and he had no intention of loving me unless I loved him back.

On reflection, what I meant when I told him that the love got in the way is that I had wanted a very formal relationship with strict discipline, and he wanted an obedient companion who did what he wanted without having to be told. I couldn't see it as a difference between what I wanted my role to be and what he wanted my role to be. I only saw it as him "doing it all wrong". I was seriously uncomfortable with him taking my feelings into account in his decisions. I wanted him to pretend I was perfect and that I was strong enough to withstand any level of harsh treatment. Of course, I'm not perfect. Pushing me too fast and too hard messed up my head. When he found that point he scaled back, gave it some time, and tried the issue from a different angle. That wasn't about love for him—it was about keeping his property functioning well and finding effective ways to get what he wanted. Loving me changed the way he felt about the decisions he made, but it didn't change the decisions.

I never stopped wanting a pure service relationship, and I still think that had things been different I could have been content and equally solidly enslaved without my master loving me. I also know that I could be fulfilled in a service-type relationship that wasn't enslavement, especially if my master was supportive of me getting that desire for total submission met through religious devotional activities. I just learned that loving and being loved is an amazing and wonderful thing that is fulfilling in an entirely different way. Keep in mind that my master found me in my early twenties, and I'd never fallen in love before. I'd had warm, affectionate feelings towards my last serious boyfriend, and I'd distantly adored the master I had prior to that, but I'd never experienced passionate love. So when I had decided I wasn't interested in a love relationship with a master (or anyone), I didn't know what I was missing.

I still think that a less emotional service relationship would be easier for me, but sometimes what's easy isn't always what's best for one's growth. I have a great deal of difficulty with appropriate emotional expression, and I am still very awkward around the whole personal-love thing, even when it's wonderful. For me, the pure service thing is about a transpersonal type of love—love of service, really, and that would make me all adoring and whatnot towards my master, and wouldn't require much emotional expression from him at all.

However, my efforts to control my emotional expression form one of my biggest walls, and I would expect (in hindsight) that any attempt to fully enslave me would likely involve taking that down. Falling madly in love for the first time was very effective at that, but whatever method was used, getting me to the point of being very emotionally expressive with my master would likely lead to me having a certain kind of deep emotional something towards him. I suppose I could be enslaved without my master dealing directly with that sort of emotional thing, but it is such an obvious target. Besides, I know I'm better suited to my master this way.

So I've made devotion to him part of my spiritual path. It's like what the Hindus refer to as the *bhakti* path, where one works toward pure and nonjudgmental love toward the Deity of your choice, only I'm applying it to him. Not that he's a deity, but he is a worthy focus to practice that spiritual devotion on.

Q: Without love, what will keep the slave safe from abuse?

Raven: Honor. Right action. Wanting to do things the right way. Wanting to be worthy of being a master. Believing that what you put out comes back to you, in one way or another. Not wanting to be merely a destructive, wasteful dickhead. But that all comes back to honor.

Love will not stop abuse. Thousands of couples batter and abuse each other, even though there may be love between them. The idea that love can keep people from hurting each other is ridiculous. If love goes away, if that's all that's holding away bad treatment, then you're in trouble. And love, being only an emotion, can get temporarily overridden by other emotions. I am emotionally capable of loving someone passionately and treating them horribly. It is my honor that keeps me treating people decently. It's stronger than my emotions, and a damn good thing too.

If there is one quality that a would-be submissive ought to look for in a dominant, in my opinion, it is honor, not love. If the owner is an honorable person, it won't matter how they feel about the slave. They will do their best to make good judgments about what will harm that slave, what will do them good and keep them going, what they can and can't endure. If an owner is indifferent but honorable, the slave will at least be safe. Actually, I think that one of the signs of someone who is trustworthy enough to own another human being is that they treat any living responsibilities with basic decency and courtesy, regardless of how they feel about them. People whose treatment of others varies depending on their emotional state are not a good choice for ownership.

Q: Does love interfere when the dominant is trying to hurt the submissive a lot in SM? Does it get in the way of sadism?

Raven: Everybody keeps bringing up the SM as the problem point for love interfering in a M/s relationship. I think that's because they don't understand that a classic sadist can hurt someone while loving them deeply, and the two are not at odds. If the dominant gets to the point of sadism where the submissive can't take it any more, stopping should be done not out of love, but out of a sense that this is the right thing to do. On the other hand, where I've found it to be a problem is when I have to make Joshua do something that I need him to do in "everyday" life that he hates and that makes him miserable. We'll cover that in the next question.

Q: If the owner forces the slave do things they don't like, doesn't that mean that they don't care about them? Or, at least, that they are totally indifferent to them as people? How can a M/s relationship be healthy if there is indifference?

Raven: This should probably best be answered by someone who is in a functioning pure-service relationship. That's a perspective that is often missed among all the lovey-dovey folks. (Among whom I am afraid I am one. But my point still stands.) But just because you make someone do something they don't like doesn't mean that you have no regard for them.

As an example: I have a barn full of sheep and goats. While the sheep are largely my housemate's project, the goats are all mine. I am not in love with my goats. They are not pets. They are livestock. They provide milk and meat. Still, I do my best to take care of them and make sure that they are as comfortable as I can make them, not because of how I feel about them, but because of how I feel about my responsibilities to living creatures in my care, be they slaves or goats. I have to do things to my goats all the time that they hate—hoof trimming, vaccinations, keeping them fenced in, making them get in the stanchion and be milked, sometimes even taking the young males out back and shooting and butchering them for meat.

I'm a parent, and I won't even go into all the things I have had to do to raise a child that the child hated. (Nearly every parent has had a moment when they told the kid that they couldn't play in the street or stick their fingers in light sockets or skip school, and the kid screamed "I hate you!" and the parent had to not let it affect them.) And, yes, sometimes I make my boy do things that he hates. Be on medication, for example. He hates that. I think it's necessary. I win. There are also many other things that he'd like to do that he can't, from

236 | RAVEN KALDERA & JOSHUA TENPENNY

cutting his hair off to taking that fun-looking college class to running off to a monastery periodically. I say he can't, because it doesn't fit in with my plans and needs, and he is made miserable for a while ... and since I love him, this makes me feel bad. Doesn't mean that I necessarily change my mind, but I'm not such a cold bastard that it doesn't affect me, if only to make me continually reevaluate how miserable I'm making him, and when I should be merciful for his mental health. This has nothing to do with sadism, it's about what's a want and what's a need.

Doing things to someone or something in your power that they hate is not a sign of indifference to them as a being. It is a sign of indifference to their (possibly irrational) desires, when you have decided that in your best judgment this is the best balance of your needs, their needs, and the realities of the situation. This is not necessarily abuse. As an owner—of humans or goats—sometimes we have to make decisions based on what we think will be best all around. My goats would probably prefer to be free to wander the neighbor's yard and rip up their rosebushes, and not to be kept for their milk. I want their milk, and I know better than them about the effect of human law on stray goats, so too bad for them. In return, I keep them healthy and give them a comparatively decent life.

It's up to the owner to decide if the unpleasant thing will really screw the slave up emotionally to do, or if they'll just hate it but be otherwise all right, or if they can find some joy in pleasing or serving even throughout the nastiness. Perhaps you've never been in the situation of having one's owner desperately want something that pains the slave terribly to give, yet the slave wants so badly to please the owner and be a good slave that they are desperate to martyr themselves for it. That's a tangle of who-gets-their-wants-met that only the owner can sort out, and then only through judgment and not knee-jerk compliance with the anyone's feelings.

People in M/s relationships have discussed how their master will not allow them to have children, or will not allow them to have Job X or Hobby Y, or expects them to adapt to non-monogamy, or whatever. When these things are discussed online on lists or forums, or in real-time in support groups, often half the listeners are saying, "Why that's abusive! How dare the owner not work hard to keep the slave happy!" and another quarter is saying, "Yup, that's just the way it is." (I think the last quarter is saying, "You mean that an owner would do that to me? Eeep!") That's where the love vs. dominance thing really comes in—how miserable are you willing to make this slave in order to get your own needs met? It's a delicate balancing act, and one that love can sometimes throw off.

And when it goes off, it goes off into the owner building up a fund of resentment and feeling less in control of the situation, and that always ends badly. Not so much of a "my slave is telling me what to do" as a "damn, whenever I want to do something my slave doesn't like, they get so fucked up that I have to stop or I'm a total crud, and maybe it's not their fault, but now I feel like I might as well be in a vanilla relationship with some kinky sex.". And, frankly, any slave whose owner always defaults to the slave's feelings rather than the owner's judgment when there is a hard choice between the two ... well. Really, who's in charge there?

Q: Do you love your slave because of who they are, or because they serve you?

Raven: I struggled with answering this one. I really wanted to give a clear answer about different kinds and levels of love ... that I can love my egalitarian wife for who she is and not for what she does for me (obviously), and that my love for my slaveboy is a different kind of love. And so forth. But I kept trying to write that and erasing it, because it wasn't the kernel of truth. That truth is that I cannot separate the two. I tried, mentally, creating all sorts of scenarios in my head about "if things were different, would I love him differently..." but it didn't work.

Joshua was submissive to me from the beginning of our relationship. Part of the reason that I took so long to accept him as my boy is that I wanted to be sure that he was suitable—and that "suitable" implied a great deal of natural submission and service-orientation. It implied that he would be a certain sort of person, right down to his core, to start with. He is not, and never has been, and would never be comfortable being, the sort of person who would not want to be submissive in relationship to me, or who would not want to serve me, instinctively.

That's the person I fell in love with. I fell in love with a natural servant, who pines when I don't find him things to do for me. The things that he does for me are part and parcel of who he is. They cannot be separated from him, and therefore I cannot separate the two. Is this falling in love with him, or with his service? The two are one. It's all the same. His urge to service is part of what made him, as a person, so easy to fall deeply in love with.

Religion and Spirituality

**Q: Should a master force a slave to convert to their religion?
Do they have the obligation to honor the slave's religion?
Should the worship of your master come before the worship of
your God(s)?**

Raven: Obviously, this question will vary depending on how
devout both the dominant and the submissive are. If the
dominant is a devout believer and the submissive isn't, the
dominant needs to decide whether or not they care if the
submissive is just going through the motions. If they don't care,
and if they are certain that their God(s) wouldn't care either,
then it doesn't seem like a problem to make the submissive
observe a particular religion. If they do care ... well, believing
religious conversion isn't something that you can just order. It
either comes or it doesn't.

The problem usually comes in when the slave is very
devout. It's the same issue regardless of whether the owner is
very devout in another faith, or a complete atheist: can they
respect the slave's religious beliefs, even when those beliefs are
inconvenient to the owner? They'll have to work out for
themselves what's too much to put up with. Differences can
arise from religiously-based ethical beliefs clashing, or the need
for particular observances becoming inconvenient, time-
consuming, and/or expensive. For myself, I believe that God(s)
trump masters, so I would find it hypocritical and spiritually
wrong to cut someone off from their religion.

I think religion is one of those slippery subjects where
everyone thinks that everything will be just fine, but then when
push comes to shove it isn't. It's hard to tell what people will
feel.

Joshua: I don't worship my master, or at least not in the
religious sense. As a devoutly religious person, I'm certain he'd
find that inappropriate. I serve the divine through my service to

my master, but that is not a substitute for giving proper reverence to the divine. However, there is a bit from the Rule of St. Benedict, on obedience:

> *This obedience, however, will be acceptable to God and agreeable to men then only if what is commanded is done without hesitation, delay, lukewarmness, grumbling or complaint, because the obedience which is rendered to Superiors is rendered to God.*

I strive to serve my master with a whole heart. That is more than just not whining—it means not complaining on the inside, either. It is not faking enthusiasm, but showing genuine enthusiasm and enjoying whatever work I am set to. I strive to be as naked and transparent with my master as I am before God, while being quite aware that he is not one.

Q: I want my slave to do something that she thinks is religiously wrong. We're both conservative Christians, but I want her to have sex with another woman for me. It's a fantasy I've had for a long time. I could order her, and force her to do it, and then it wouldn't be her fault; she would just be following orders. At least that's what I tell her, but she isn't willing to sin on my order. How can I get her comfortable enough with that lack of responsibility?

Raven: I'm an owner who is strongly religious, and I have a very religious slave. In my opinion, either the owner respects the slave's religion (regardless of whether they believe in it) or they don't. Forcing a slave to do something that goes against their religion is a clear communication from the owner that no, they do not respect the slave's religion, and they feel free to violate it whenever the whim takes them. Assuming that the slave actually believes that X action is Wrong for religious reasons, and that there Will Be Consequences for indulging in it—consequences doled out by a higher power than the master, and thus not in the master's power to protect the slave from—then this can be a disaster.

Were I to order my slave to do something against his faith, I would expect him to: A) understand that I have no respect for the strength of his religious beliefs and his deep spiritual needs, B) understand that I do not care if he believes that there will be spiritual consequences for that act, and C) think much, much less of me as a person.

I'm queer as a three-dollar bill, and I'm Pagan, and I don't believe that queerness is wrong, duh. But ... I know what conservative Christian people believe, even if I may personally feel that it is inaccurate. I also know that the key that holds this belief in place is fear of punishment from God. It isn't just about guilt. If it's just a vague sense of guilt, not a real fear of God, then they aren't really all that deeply religious—they just may be holding to a cultural religious viewpoint, and whether the owner ought to muck with that is up to their own sense of ethics.

If I thought that a slave was in the second category—say, just holding to a cultural religious viewpoint more out of habit than anything else—I might try to work on them regarding the more undesirable parts of it. I might do that by introducing them to devout people of their faith whose "take" on their religion approved of the parts that I found convenient or true, and had dispensed with the ones that I found undesirable, and encourage the slave to talk to them about it. Or I might take that job on myself—not breaking them of their faith, but showing them that there are many ways to live that faith.

If I had a slave who was entirely devout, and willing to put their beliefs ahead of me, perhaps for reasons of saving their immortal soul ... well, Gods trump masters, and that's that. I would not disrespect their beliefs in that way. If those beliefs got in the way of my will so badly as to cause me massive and frustrating inconvenience, then I suppose we wouldn't be suited to each other and we should call it quits (and as the owner, that's my responsibility to realistically decide). There's no shame in deciding that this simply isn't going to work out.

But, basically, it comes down to this for a slave who is caught between a religious belief and their master's orders: Are you more afraid of defying your Higher Power and your spiritual path, or defying your master? If you're in the former category, you'll defy your master and hold to your beliefs, no matter what—and your Higher Power will give you that strength, no matter how owned you are, possibly breaking the master's hold on you if necessary. If you're more afraid of your dominant than God, then you're not really all that religious.

Q: When I hear talk about submissives giving up their desires, it sounds a lot like what religious mystics go through. Is it that similar? And what is the spiritual counterpart of that quest for the dominant?

Joshua: It is indeed very similar, or it can be. Even submissives who aren't very spiritual to start with can suddenly find themselves describing their experience of deep submission in terms that sound a lot like a mystic on an ascetic path. Spirituality can sneak up on a slave in that way. After all, it is a path of letting go, giving up the ego and the "small-S self", learning to be adaptable to any hardship, and searching for serenity in serving others. Some religions stress this as the ideal path for everyone. I don't think this is true, but it certainly is my path.

I have a very strong monastic streak. Life as a monk gives you very little free will, and that isn't at all scary or unpleasant to me. It never was. Surrendering the will is a valuable lesson, a way of taming your ego. It is too easy to get caught up in satisfying your own whims, and too easy to form a definition of "self" based on trivial preferences. Having this stripped away is actually very liberating. I would much rather be subject to my master's will than to my own petty emotional drives.

Raven: We dominants have our own self-perfecting that we need to work on, but we are not going to be perfectly confident, perfectly organized, perfectly patient, perfectly introspective, and never erring in judgment just because we've had a slave for a few months or a year. We, too, are a work in progress, and our end-goal—should we choose to go that route—is just as difficult to achieve.

In my mind, from a spiritual perspective at least, if my slave is going to struggle to give up all his desires and values (in a very Zen-like way) and take on all of mine, then mine had better be well-scrutinized and as close to the point of perfection as I can humanly make them, in order for those values and desires to be worthy of taking on the "karma", if you will, of two people. So there is, ideally, struggle and continual work on both sides. There will also be mistakes, procrastination, prevarication, backsliding, and general stupidity on both sides, because we are flawed humans. But that's part of the deal.

Q: I've heard it said that it's the Owner's responsibility to make the slave's personal development a high priority, as part of doing M/s as a spiritual path. Yet at the same time, I thought that the Owner's desires are supposed to come first? Which is it? How does one balance that out?

Raven: I've written before about how much of slave ownership is a delicate balancing act, a conscious strategizing between what one desires, what one can realistically have, and what one should be doing in order to do the right thing. It's a back-and-forth. Doing the right moral, ethical, whatever-you-call-it thing, for me, does require that I put effort into my slave's personal development. (This goes above and beyond simply not harming him; it's pushing him to do self-improvement things that he would not have done on his own semi-lazy will, and which actively inconvenience me.) What I may desire is entirely selfish and would probably pull in the opposite direction. Those two poles must be balanced. What I can realistically have, given the limitations of we two flawed human beings, is the boundary around that tug-of-war.

So one starts with the things that work for both. How can I improve him in ways that will have clear benefits for me? Helping him to make lists and become more organized is a minor inconvenience, but it results in a better-functioning houseboy. Sending him to school for massage was a big inconvenience, but it gave him both a flexible service-oriented career and a skill that I can now enjoy for the rest of my life. In this case, the inconvenience was worth it, and that's what I told my grumbling selfish self while it was going on. It "proves" to that selfish side of me that it is worth the trouble.

After doing a good deal of that, I have slowly started dipping toes here and there into specific areas of his improvement that have no actual direct benefit for me. Why bother? Well, first because it is the right thing to do. One could say that this is me making a commitment not to my slave, but to my own code of honor. One could also say that my self-image is strongly bound up with my code of honor, and so I do myself good when I do occasional entirely unselfish things. I'm also a Maker, a Crafter, and I take a certain amount of satisfaction in improving my property for the sake of improving it, just as I would polish a piece of craftwork.

However, I have to be careful with myself. I notice that when I go too far off the path of direct benefits for too long—when too much of my limited resources get channeled into improving my slave for no direct benefit—the selfish, irrational part of me acts up and says, "Wait a minute. Who's in charge here? Who's supposed to be the one Getting Their Way in this relationship after all?" Then I have to back off and be more selfish, less altruistic with him. Why feed that? Because it's the selfish part of my soul that contributes that visceral feeling of ownership for both of us, and without that I might as well just be a boss, therapist, or life coach. The rational part of me can be responsible, be fair, be ethical, be practical, be introspective, be appraising, be honorable. The irrational part of me Owns, deeply and powerfully in a way that he responds to strongly.

How else can I put this? The clenched fist in the hair, the growl—"You are mine." The feeling, the rush that accompanies this. His body responds to mine, saying, "Yes, I am yours," and the barrier is broken down. Then the rational part of me can get in there and do its various things with him. But the Beast must be fed and pacified, for although it must be kept in check, its job is crucial. If you don't feel like you own them, they can tell, and it all goes downhill from there. So it's a balancing game.

> *"I would have you consider your judgment and your appetite even as you would two loved guests in your house. Surely you would not honour one guest above the other; for he who is more mindful of one loses the love and the faith of both." -Kahlil Gibran*

Q: Doesn't being a slave mean that you have to sacrifice important things in your future?

Raven: Yes, it does, which is why it is not something to be taken on without a great deal of thought. To illustrate this, I want to mention something which has had Joshua in tears a few times. He has a strong call to monasticism, and the ways in which slavery resembles monasticism are very good for him. However, since he is permanently in service to me until I'm dead, he will not actually be able to enter a monastery and take vows until after my death. Since I'm older than him and in poor health, it's quite likely that he'll get there eventually, but sometimes he pines for the idea.

He had a bit of a weeping fit about it once, and I encouraged him to do his prayer beads nightly, and to read more on monasticism. Then we talked about the monastic issue of vows of stability. That's the vow that keeps the monk from deciding that maybe that monastery over there would be better than this one, or that one, or that one—it encourages them to commit to one place and work on their stuff rather than trying to escape it by running about. He came, quickly and on his own, to the realization that this was advice relevant to his commitment here—that when living a narrow, disciplined spiritual path, it is better to commit to one place and set of vows and try to work it out than to constantly obsess about all the things you can't do if you're doing something else.

(He has also had problems in the past with my low-protocol approach, and it was helpful for him to read about new monks who complained that their Order was more lax than they dreamed of, and asked for more austerities to pile on them, and the abbot gently suggests that they get to doing the existing austerities perfectly and with a better attitude before whining for more. It's amazing how much wisdom the Benedictines and the Buddhists have for slaves.)

But realistically, this isn't just limited to slaves. There are things that I will never do because of the commitments I've made. Every time you commit to anything, a hundred other possibilities die. That's life. The only way to avoid that is to live commitmentless, and nobody ever accomplished anything of worth that way. You can't have focus without limits, you can't have shape without pruning.

Joshua: It is a very difficult and interesting question because there are so many ways to read it. For instance, since we walk the path of spiritual service and mastery, by doing service in the context of this relationship, sacrifice becomes an act of spiritual devotion. The submission sanctifies the service. As to my own spiritual path, I was never the sort who wanted to change the world. I had no ambition; I was quite content with my place in things. I'm a cog, you know? That was fine with me. I never felt a strong desire to "make something" of myself, though for a while I thought I was terribly flawed because of that. Entering into service with my master meant that all of a sudden I was part of larger goals—his goals. This has been amazing to me.

But you're probably wondering: Don't you miss your personal agency when it's connected to something that's really important to you? Deeply, and one of those things has had me in tears before, as my master has pointed out. But this here is my life—service to my master—and that is just the way of it. This is the best use of me as far as the universe is concerned, and in my heart I know that. That means there are some things I will never do, and some things that cannot happen while I am in service to my master, and some things that I will only be able to touch the edges of. It is painful, but that's part of any life that you give yourself over to fully. My master told me that there is an old Romany proverb that goes, "With one butt you cannot ride two horses." Yeah, that's the way of things.

Many of the things I might be tempted to call sacrifices are more what I'd call compromises, though I don't mean compromises between my master and I. I mean situations where you want A and B, but can't have both. If you take A, does that mean not taking B was a sacrifice? If so, there are many sacrifices in my life. I walk a narrow path, and there are many things I feel called to that I cannot have/do/be, things that were sacrificed in favor of my path of service to my master. I cannot quite say that I have made these sacrifices, because my role in the choosing is debatable, but I will say that sacrifices have been made—by my master, by Fate, by the Powers that Be, and perhaps by me as well.

Once in a while it becomes very painful to think about the life I would have had, or could have had, if I had not been given to my master. I look at the space where that life would have been, and I mourn its loss. I don't regret it, or resent it, but I do mourn it from time to time. But hey, limitations are part of the price for embodied existence. I can only live one life, and it may be that whatever life I had, I'd mourn the ones I didn't. In any case, while my life was sacrificed for my master, in my day-to-day service I don't feel like I am making continual sacrifices. I am just living my life.

In some ways, this conversation can bring out the same issues as the "gift of submission" debate, and highlights the distinction between giving out of obligation, being compelled to give, giving on a whim of one's one free will, and giving what one is obligated to give with an open heart.

Q: I'm submissive, a would-be slave, with a strong spiritual vocation in my life. I want to be in a power dynamic relationship very badly, but only with a dominant who I can respect as my spiritual superior. The dominant I'm talking to right now isn't as far ahead on their path as I am on mine, and I don't know if I can respect them enough to be owned by them. What can I do?

Raven: With more and more people discovering D/s and M/s as spiritual paths, and wanting to incorporate them into their lives in that way, we see this question more and more. Sometimes it's asked to us directly, as in the above amalgamate quote, and sometimes we're helping to counsel a couple about their power dynamic and we discover this is really what's going on.

While we've met people on both sides of the dynamic who are strongly connected to spirituality, there definitely seems to be a surplus on the submissive side, at least for now. That may be because the very nature of submission can force you into a spiritual place you didn't expect, whereas the mastery path requires more active pursuing and solitary struggle and is harder to inadvertently fall into. There's also a lot less information about it out there, and dominants are less willing to talk about their sensitive issues in public, leaving newer dominants with no signposts. This means that until the numbers even out, there are going to be a lot more submissives in this predicament.

While integrating your power exchange into your spiritual path is not something that all couples are going to want to do (and there's no reason that they must; there's nothing inherently wrong with ethical but nonspiritual relationships), those of us who have found this path are often "spoiled", as it were, for relationships without it. I can speak from experience that finding the right spiritual path outside of your relationships can be so huge and all-encompassing that it colors everything else. Having the relationship structure be part of that path can so completely change your expectations that relating without it can be impossibly unfulfilling. For those who are called to this path, it can in its own way be compared to going back to an egalitarian vanilla relationship after the intensity of SM and power exchange.

Joshua: It is really tough to balance a spiritual calling with 24/7 service when the dominant isn't part of that calling. Both are roles that will expand to fill whatever container you are able to provide for them, and both have a tendency to overfill what you can comfortably offer. There often isn't room in anyone's life for two such demanding containers, which is why it works so much better when both are mixed.

When subs tell us that their dominant is "not at as high a level" as they are spiritually, it can mean a lot of different things. It could mean "not as far along in his spiritual development as me" or "not as invested in her spiritual beliefs or practices as I am" or even, in some cases, "I'm in a position of spiritual authority over my dominant in the same spiritual church or tradition." Whatever the situation, it's hard.

I think it is very, very challenging for a deeply spiritual person to submit fully to someone who isn't their spiritual superior (or at least their equal) in some meaningful way. For one thing, when things come to a difficult place in the D/s, it is tempting to play the "God card" and put your spirituality between you and the dominant. If they have to defer entirely to your judgment on that, it can undermine the development of real power exchange.

It's also much easier when both people have a similar understanding about following one's spiritual path, and can commiserate and help each other through. That's useful for couples regardless of power dynamics, but it's especially useful when the dominant must make informed decisions about the sub's life that may impact their practices. And, of course, some subs have a strong need for the "disciple's path" as part of their relational archetypes, and must have a master who is not only strongly spiritual but someone that they can look up to as a spiritual superior. Others simply need someone who is as spiritually dedicated and committed as they are, and can equally shoulder the burden of integrating the relationship into the path.

It's worse if the reverse happens, of course, with the D/s protecting the sub from some challenging aspect of their spiritual path. When you have a genuine calling, anything you let get in the way can be taken from you, no matter how painful it is. Announcing to the Universe that you're going to make your spiritual path a priority means that the Universe is going to take you seriously on that, and putting a relationship first will doom that relationship. The D/s or M/s bond must at the least harmonize with your path, and ideally serve it.

Earlier in this book, I spoke about emotional takedowns and not allowing the field where the slave excels to become the main field of importance for the relationship. The one area where this rule doesn't work is spirituality, for the reasons outlined in the last paragraph. A submissive whose life is bound up with their spiritual path to the point where they can't serve a human being who isn't out there with them … should probably pray to the Powers That Be to provide them with the right partner, and not settle for less, for their own psychic well-being.

Lifestyle Variations:
Who, What, and Where

Gender Roles

Q: What are your roles like, compared to vanilla roles? How are they affected by the fact that you're a same-sex couple?

Joshua: In many ways, I'm very much a housewife. I've had women ask me if my master's wife resents me taking "her job". I laugh. His wife keeps house about as well as your average frat boy, and she's never considered housekeeping to be "her job". Also, my master and I have a professional relationship that often overshadows the romantic relationship. I'm mostly expected to be productive and Do My Job, not just be a homemaker and fun-time companion.

I think that what makes it more of a "traditional marriage" dynamic than a male/male hierarchy is that there is no sense of room for advancement. In many gay leather households there is such a concept, with some portion of the men making a progression from slave to master after sufficient experience. There is a sense from the master that he was once in the slave's place, and therefore knows how to bring the slave to a level of development where he could theoretically be a master in his own right. If you are looking at the military, or management positions in a corporation, there is that same idea of working your way through the ranks. A parent-child or student-teacher relationship has something similar. In a mobile hierarchy there is an inequality of role, but not an inequality of fundamental nature.

A traditional husband-wife dynamic is a static hierarchy. Young wives grow up to be old wives, and young husbands to be old husbands, with no progression between roles. Traditional race/ethnicity based service/slavery systems fall into this category, as does any strongly caste-based hierarchy. There are complex inter-group hierarchies with a certain amount of mobility, but there is no moving from one group to the other. A slavery framework where masters and slaves are seen as having fundamentally differing natures would be another example, regardless of whether the roles are believed to be gendered.

Raven: One's roles in a power dynamic can be influenced by many things—traditional heterosexual roles, pornography, historical roles, various leather cultures, the military, religious faiths, or even fantasy novels. That said, we've certainly seen people in M/s relationships both clinging to "traditional" roles and doing things entirely differently. It does seem to be easier for male-dominant/female-submissive couples to "default" to something that looks like a 1950s housewife model, complete with the strong accent on monogamy, but some innovative folks eschew this and copy other models. Gay M/s relationships also tend in the majority toward a model somewhere between military discipline and servant/houseboy, and a significant percentage of lesbian M/s relationships copy the gay model.

We've seen female-dominant/male-submissive couples that fall into the "porn model" of queenly (and often mean) dominatrix who uses and thinks little of her humiliated male slave (or slaves; this version is often nonmonogamous because there's an assumption that the femme-domme neither has sex with nor is emotionally attached to her men) but that role tends to be short-term. When we've seen long-term romantic female-dominant/male-submissive couples, they have almost always dispensed with the porn roles and created something else.

While the "something elses" in many of these examples are all unique, we do notice that they often entirely dispense with any kind of gendered behavior, regardless of gender combinations.

Q: What about gender-crossing individuals in power dynamic relationships? Are there are patterns evident in the way that they choose to identify?

Raven: It's been fascinating to be privileged to watch so many transsexuals and other transgendered individuals navigate the waters of power exchange. Watching a large and varied number of such folks up close and personal with their D/s and M/s choices definitely puts the lie to the idea of "naturally gendered" D/s. Sometimes it's by watching the anomalies that you get the real information about the study. For example, in the theories of "naturally gendered" D/s, should transsexuals fall into the category of their birth gender or the one that they transitioned to? (Of course, I've unfortunately found that most of the proponents of "naturally gendered" M/s simply tend to prefer that transfolks didn't exist.)

The actual truth is that transsexuals are all over the map. Some are dominant and some are submissive (and some are switches), in fairly equal numbers regardless of what gender they started or ended in. Some stay the same regardless of their transition, and some switch over once they transition.

Of course, they also cite social pressures as being as much of a factor as their own natural (and widely varied) power exchange proclivities. One FTM (female-to-male) transsexual we know was raised in a traditional family, and told that women had to be submissive; he was unhappily submissive throughout his female life and could only become happily dominant once he changed over. Another FTM was raised to believe that women should be strongly independent, and could only settle contentedly into being a submissive houseboy once he'd become male and would no longer be a "politically non-transgressive" housewife. One MTF (male-to-female transsexual) that we know thought that she would have to be submissive because that was part of her cultural understanding of femaleness and something she'd eroticized; after transition and a lowering of libido, she discovered that she was more comfortable maintaining her culturally-taught masculine dominance even while being female, and became her partner's queenly domme. Another MTF discovered contented submission after becoming a woman ... and so on. There's no overriding pattern for people who've been and lived both, and this in itself is telling.

(If there is one thing that we've noticed as a high statistic, it's the small observation that when FTMs go sub, they're almost always very service-oriented instead of being mainly control-oriented. We are not sure of statistics in other directions, and even this may merely be a product of our sample set. Rather than looking at gender sorted by D/s, perhaps it might be more interesting to look at gender sorted by service vs. control? Or not.)

Q: I'm transgendered, and I'm having a hard time finding a dominant. Recently, a dom contacted me, but when I found out that he's a crossdresser, I turned him down. Why can't I get a real man or woman as a dom?

Raven: So what's wrong with having a dominant who's also transgendered?

I know that transfolk, especially transsexuals, are the only cultural subcategory who are openly discouraged from dating each other by the "gatekeepers". Transfolk are told that you aren't "real", you haven't validated your gender, unless you have a "real"—meaning single-gendered—partner. It used to be "heterosexual single partner"; now it's slid a little to allow for gay/lesbian relationships, but dating each other is still considered "cheating" on some weird level.

I think this is garbage. I also think that it's unhealthy. Who can better understand the issues of a TG slave than a TG master? Let's face it, no matter how much a single-gendered person may love you and/or study you, there are going to be certain things that they simply won't get. Period. That doesn't mean that it can't work, but a TG owner definitely has the advantage there. So the question is... why are you biased against a TG owner? Especially when you seem to be unhappy about potential owners being biased against you as a TG slave?

You might want to think about how much of the above unhealthy attitude you may have absorbed. You might also want to think hard about whether you hope for a non-TG partner (D/s or not) in order to validate your gender in some way. ("I must be a girl—a straight man wants me in spite of my genitalia!") That's unfair. No lover should exist to validate your gender. Only you can do that.

The hard truth, which isn't your fault at all, is that most people do not want TG folks as lovers. Part of that is sexual preference—unless they're at least partly bisexual, they're going to want one or the other. Partly because they don't know what to do with TG lovers; there isn't enough positive and realistic TG erotica out there to give people a context. (Although some of us are working on it!) Partly it's fear of being with someone so "different".

So as a slave, this is a definite problem in your "price on the block", as it were. In one of the books in Laura Antoniou's *Marketplace* series, the FTM transsexual trainer Chris Parker—who wants to be a slave—tells about how he became a trainer instead because he thinks that no one would want him as a slave now that he's become what he wanted. It's rough, and I sympathize. Knowing that becoming the person that you really are, instead of living a lie all your life, will make people less likely to want to form relationships with you, is a hard and unfair thing. I wish it was different, and I hope to see change on that front as the decades progress. But you are doing yourself no favors to turn down potential partners for the same traits that others turn you down for.

It may be that you associate transgenderedness with submission. (I know a few transgendered submissives who somehow got that strange idea in their head, especially if they conflated cross-gender fantasies with submissive fantasies in their youth.) Boy, is that something that you need to get over! Some of the meanest "dragon lady" dommes that I know are MTFs, and some of the toughest leather daddies that I know are FTMs. The cross-dressing dom who talked to you ... can you imagine his female side as all your best and worst Dragon Lady fantasies rolled into one package—and then tomorrow, he can be a man and dominate you in an entirely different way? Honey, this is *not* a disadvantage!

Or ... does it scare you, the idea of being owned by someone who knows, intimately, exactly what all your dysphoria feels like ... and can reach into you and use that, with a much more knowing hand than that longed-for single-gendered straight partner? Heh. Something to think about. If your blood runs cold at the idea, I think you'd better wait on looking to be enslaved.

Q: I'm a MtF cross-dresser, living with my master. I am planning to start hormones soon, so that I can become the woman of his dreams. Is there anything that I need to know before I begin?

Raven: You and your master need to know this:

While there is a continuum of transgenderism—from occasional sexually-driven transvestitism to full-on non-sexual primary transsexualism—if you are dealing with libido-driven urges, you have to be careful how far you go. In other words, if your attraction to this is mostly sexual—and there's nothing wrong with that, we all have fetishes—if your libido is reduced, it may cease to be any fun for you.

The application of estrogen often decreases libido drastically, and operations that remove the testes make that even more serious. Indeed, one of the biggest sexual problems of post-transition male-to-female transsexuals is sheer lack of sex drive ... because sex drive, in both men and women, is testosterone-driven. I've seen this happen before, multiple times ... someone still living in the male role is terribly turned on by the idea of being feminized and/or living as a woman and/or getting a female body; they go further and further with it until they decide to start taking estrogen (perhaps they want breasts, soft skin, other female cues) and then the bottom falls out. Their libido declines, and the hard-on that was making it all so sexy isn't there any more. Generally one of two things happens:

1) They realize that they are really male-to-female transsexuals, and the eroticism of it was just their subconscious mind feeding it out through the libido in order to get their attention about their repressed urges. They go on with transition and live full-time as women, but there's nothing sexual about it any more, it's just what's for breakfast. The whole cross-dressing/sissy/feminization thing isn't sexy any more ... and they get to deal with the issue of possibly lowered libido. On the other hand, they may be happier, calmer, and more fulfilled in terms of their all-around life. Generally they consider it all worth it, even if they aren't much of a pervert any more. It's emotional satisfaction instead of sexual satisfaction.

2) The attraction to the sissy/feminization thing vanishes, because their attraction to everything is lessened, and it doesn't seem interesting any more, and they quit. (Actually, if wanting to be a slave is primarily sexual for you, that will go out the window too.) As soon as the testosterone is back up, so are the fetishes. I know people who struggled with this for years—when they were off estrogen, they wanted to be women, and desperately wanted to take it in order to feminize themselves. When they went on estrogen, they ceased to want to be women, and didn't care any more.

So you'll have to be careful if your master intends to muck with your endocrine system. Just a warning.

Polyamory and M/s

Q: What about when a master wants more than one slave? I'm terrified that if I give up power in a relationship, the dominant would decide to take on another girl, and then I'd be heartbroken. Does a slave have the right to require that her master be monogamous?

Raven: You're asking a polyamory question, and whether that works strongly depends on whether the slave in question is OK with being polyamorous or not. Even the most dedicated slave is still human, and if they would not be comfortable with polyamory in a vanilla relationship, that doesn't change just because they get owned. On the other hand, really-truly-owned slaves sometimes end up poly whether they like it or not, because yes, they give up the right to decide who will be sexually exclusive with whom, or to have any control over their partner's bits. I think that this is especially difficult for monogamously-inclined submissives in romantic relationships with their partners, who have a starry-eyed idea that this will be in many ways like a vanilla bodice-ripper except kinkier.

Whether the s-type has the "right" to demand that their owner be monogamous depends on how many rights they are allowed, and how absolute the dynamic is. In some arrangements, the slave has no rights, but must depend on the dominant's honor and the promises that they have made. In less absolute dynamics, the submissive has the right to enforce monogamy, or at least to walk out if it isn't upheld. Interestingly enough, forced polyamory does seem to be the single most frequent subject for so many (especially female) submissives to be laying down very unsubmissive lines about. I hear "If my Master decided not to be monogamous with me, I'd leave him (or throw a fit or whatever)" far, far more often than I hear stuff about physically damaging behavior or moral issues or whatever. It really seems to haunt the thoughts of many submissives.

I think it's because polyamory is an ambivalent ethical issue. Activities that involve endangering the physical health of the sub, or clearly immoral issues (making the sub steal or kill for you), well, those are going to be weighed in on as "bad" by nearly everyone. But many people think that polyamory is perfectly fine, that there's nothing inherently wrong with it, as long as everyone involved has given consent. And with an owned slave, well, they've already given up a lot of their right to consent to things, so how do polyamory rules work then?

There's a huge grey area around D/s and polyamorous protocol (which is why when I wrote my book on polyamory, I left out the entirety of the D/s question, as it would have muddied the waters and probably needed its own entire book). People don't have a good, clear, community-accepted model to turn to, as most of the people in the poly demographic don't like or understand D/s (and so many of their rules don't apply to people without full agency), and the BDSM demographic is largely still uncomfortable with total M/s, so people are floundering. The usual rules of polyamorous consent go out the window when one person has given up their right to consent. (I'm currently working on a book with Christina Parker on just this subject—power exchange in polyamory—called *Power Circuits*, which hopefully will shed some more light on this tricky subject.)

There's another layer to this which is probably even more frightening to many subs. People change, including dominants. People's wants and needs change, and they come to learn more about themselves. Sometimes that means that the most consistent and dependable dominant will suddenly discover that they like something that they didn't think they ever would ... and I've seen that thing be polyamory so many times that it's not funny.

No, I'm not saying that every dominant who promised monogamy to their sub at the beginning, before the collar went on and the enslavement started, is going to suddenly change their mind and start realizing that they would really prefer to be polyamorous 15 years down the road. Certainly not; some people are monogamous because that's what suits them best. But some are monogamous for other reasons, reasons that don't suit them and that they may eventually discard, and that's frightening to the sub who wants everything set in stone at the beginning of the relationship, never to change, especially after they no longer have any recourse. Of course that's frightening. Giving yourself to someone else is a huge act of trust.

And yet ... it happens. People change. Dominants change, and as I said polyamory is one of the more frequent ways that I've seen them change ... and what's the slave with the desperate need for monogamy to do? The hard truth is that it's the dominant's job to do whatever it takes to slowly lead them into a place of being OK with that, and it's also true that many dominants do not have the experience or the wherewithal to do that, and that's hard on the sub. But I think that every slave needs to understand that they are taking a leap of faith, and that their dominant may change in the future.

In fact, I think that there ought to be part of the pre-claiming negotiations that sounds like, "So I know that you're swearing that everything you like now you'll always like and everything you don't want now you'll never want. But what if that changes after I'm collared? What will you do to help me be all right with that? Because just ordering me to like it and telling me that I'm a lousy slave if I can't manage that is not going to be terribly effective."

I know that's an area where most people don't want to tread—it's like being a vanilla couple and saying, "So on the off chance that we get divorced, can you convince me that you'd be a kind and reasonable ex?" Everyone wants to pretend that this never happens ... but it does, and it takes a brave couple to look at that before the commitment of whatever kind happens.

Q: I'm a dominant, and I really feel like I want to explore polyamory, but my slave is extremely insecure about the idea. There's another submissive that I'm interested in, and who is interested in possibly becoming our third, but I'm afraid that my sub will freak out. But aren't I the one in charge here?

Raven: Yes, you are the one in charge, and as such the responsibility for minimizing damage is entirely on you. First, you have to determine whether your slave is going to be able to emotionally handle your nonmonogamy. Some can't, especially if they have massive insecurity issues. In that case, you should be working on your slave's self-esteem first. Tools function better when they feel good about themselves.

There are some standard pieces of polyamorous wisdom that apply to everyone, even M/s couples. The first, and biggest one, is that you don't take on a new lover if your primary relationship is having problems. Ironically, it's an appallingly common reason to do so, but it's the worst thing you can do for either your old lover or a new one. It's actually a serial-monogamy custom ("My relationship isn't so good any more, I'll just go find a new one") rather than a polyamorous one. This means that if your submissive cannot handle a polyamorous relationship without severe emotional stress, you have only a few choices. You can remain monogamous, out of respect for their issues. You can dismiss them, and find someone more suitable to your poly needs. The only other option is that you can require them to work on the issue—something that an egalitarian partner does not have as an option—and find out if there's a way that they can be made content with the situation.

This last option is not guaranteed, and if it fails, you're back to the other two. It's also not something that they can do alone. In fact, the more help the dominant gives them, the more likely it is to succeed. That includes hour after hour of emotional processing, making small moves, constant reassurance, and a huge amount of communication between all parties, including the old slave and the new slave. If the two don't want to talk, it's up to the dominant to make them sit down and hash it out.

One of the few advantages to such a situation is that the master/mistress really can force the slaves to communicate ... but they have to put on their dominant panties and do it. One of the most common errors I've seen is a dominant who runs out, gets another lover, and then sits around covertly hoping that the two will somehow miraculously start communicating and liking each other, but ducks and evades when the stresses start taking people in the opposite direction. All too often, it's done out of fear of confrontation ("...they'll outnumber me, and they'll both start crying, and then maybe one will threaten to leave!"), or fear of losing the new nookie, or a vain and cowardly hope that it will just all work itself out. Sometimes it does, miraculously, but it's just as likely to all go wrong. Dominants who are introducing polyamory to an existing M/s relationship have to be proactive and take both control and responsibility from the beginning.

In the end, it's about trust. Even a slave who thinks that they will be fine with polyamory sometimes ends up with issues and insecurities when faced with the real thing. In order for them to feel safe, they must trust the dominant to help them get through the rough parts with as little pain as possible. If the dominant does not act and do something constructive when problems arise, the slave's trust fails yet more. It's crucial to be in control of the situation, and that means being willing to make hard decisions and be a uniting force in the face of emotional divisions.

In the meantime, the first step might be to have the slave read books on how polyamory is done, and done right. The step that follows that should probably be to have them sit down and talk with a variety of long-term polyamorous families. The ideal would be families with D/s dynamics, or who are at least kinky, but if that's not available then vanilla polyamorous folks will still have useful things to say, especially about coping with jealousy, possessiveness, territoriality, envy, and all those monsters. The dominant also needs to read up and talk to people, because the dominant needs to have an even better idea of how a healthy polyamorous situation should go, being as they will have to successfully orchestrate a delicate situation. The submissive need only learn enough to be reassured, but the dominant will be making sure that the rest of the people involved do it right.

Most D/s people who don't have much experience with polyamory tend to imagine it as being one dominant with a "stable" of submissives, but in actuality the range of variety in kinky polyamorous families is huge. As well as the aforementioned situation, there are paired (and occasionally unpaired) dominants who share one or more submissives, slaveowners with vanilla partners, hierarchies with people at the top and bottom and switches in the middle, and even submissives with a vanilla partner and a dominant. There is also great variety in the levels of D/s between relationships with any given partner; a dominant might have one egalitarian lover, one full-time slave, one full-time submissive with significantly more rights and limits, and a part-time sub that they see occasionally. Many ongoing polyamorous families end up looking more like constellations than simple geometric forms.

Q: Are you all living together in a group M/s situation? How does that work out?

Raven: I live with Joshua, with whom I am in a M/s dynamic, and my wife, with whom I have an egalitarian relationship. We live together on the same farm with two housemates, and the three of us all sleep in the same bed. However, we are not all three involved in a D/s relationship. My wife is not interested in being submissive to me (and thus she shouldn't have to), and she has no authority over Joshua just because she is married to me.

She knows that we're in this relationship, although she rather sees it as an elaborate game that we're playing. She had no problem with Joshua moving in; we've been poly for all 15 years of our marriage and she generally likes him as a person. The polyamory is not a problem.

Her initial big discomfort with the situation was a worry that having someone to wait on me would make me lazy and entitled, and that I wouldn't do my share of the housework. Living in a group house means that we have to act as if we are independent adults in terms of handing out chores; just because I have a slave doesn't mean that I can just order him to do my stuff for me all the time, because the other housemates see that as an unfair advantage. So I may be the only master who does shifts washing dishes and doing laundry, for the sake of domestic harmony. (Something that often makes other owners who live alone with their slave cross their eyes in disbelief.) And it also reassures my wife that I am not letting slaveownership make me into a tyrant or a couch potato.

Since my disabling disease has progressed, however, and Joshua now does the PCA/nursing for me (which would drive her nuts), she's happy with the fact that I have someone to take care of me physically. It's easier to have a slave to drive you around, take you to health care appointments, cook you special food, get up with you in the middle of the night when you're ill again, than to pay professionals to live in and deal with it. Since we don't have a lot of money, I couldn't afford that anyway, so we all see Joshua as a health necessity for me.

Also, since Joshua works and supports me, she can spend her own income as she pleases and not have to support me, which always made her uncomfortable. That means that we don't argue over money like we used to, so it's less stress on the marriage. So is not having to depend on her for kinky sex she doesn't want to have.

Joshua: My master's marriage to his wife predates me by more than a decade, and we've all lived together for around six years.

She is not the slightest bit submissive to my master, though she does enjoy strictly recreational BDSM play. I am polite and helpful to her, but she has no direct authority over me. (We tried that years ago, but she disagreed continually with my master about what I ought to be doing.)

As far as insecurity goes, I have never been left any doubt as to which of my master's needs I am and am not fulfilling. If he were to get a slave that met his needs in places where I fall short of the mark, I would be very thankful. It might be painful to be reminded of areas where I am struggling, but those are issues I would need to get over whether there was another slave or not. It is not my job to fulfill all of my masters needs. It is my job to serve him to the best of my ability. I have learned what happens when I lament my "failings" and doubt my worthiness of my master ... he ignores me or tells me to knock it off. "You won't be able to wash any dishes with your hands nailed to that cross, boy."

Q: What about when an owner wants their slave to have sex with someone not of their preference? I don't think that I could get it up if my owner wanted me to fuck a woman.

Raven: So who says that a penis is necessary to satisfy a woman? (Or a man?) Or for that matter, a mere flesh penis? True, some women (or men) might not have any use for a man who wasn't using a flesh penis, but then they might also prefer a man who was blond or well-built or young or tattooed or whatever. Personal tastes are not the same across the board.

My boy prefers men, but I have had him sexually satisfy people of various genders. The deal that I have with him is that nobody touches anything between his legs but me. If he's going to have sex with someone, I lock him into a chastity harness. (If they have a problem with this, and aren't interested unless they can have access to his bits, then I politely suggest that they should look elsewhere. There are plenty of genitals out there, if that's all they want.) His chastity harness has an attachment for a strap-on, and he has access to a wide variety of dildoes, so if anyone—female or male—wants him to fuck them with a phallic object, they can pick one. Otherwise, he is very good with hands and mouth. He's a former sex worker and trained professional.

This has nothing to do with his sexual preferences. You do not have to be attracted to someone to give them good professional sexual service. In fact, the fact that his genitals are not involved and he will get no physical release from the situation just makes it more of a service experience. It's not about him, or his arousal or lack of it. It's about them getting done properly, if the way in which they want to get done is something that he can provide.

Any slave who uses a lack of attraction for a reason not to have sex with someone on their owner's command is missing the point. You'd sweep their floor if your owner ordered it, yes? You'd rub their feet? You'd take out their trash? Sex under those circumstances is no different. If you can't make the plumbing go up, that's a physical problem, like not being able to take out their trash that day because your ankle was sprained. The owner should understand that your plumbing might not work, but your fingers and mouth aren't broken, right? And your hole(s), if you're allowed to use them.

Really, what's usually going on is a struggle for identity. People's sexual preference is part of how they define themselves, and what observers see them do is part of how they define that preference. It isn't enough to simply know in your heart that you are Preference X, even if you are having sex with someone different from that; most people worry that if they sleep "outside" their preference, everyone will think that they're not really what they say they are. To be ordered to sexually service someone outside your preference is a way for the dominant to say, "Your identity is what I say it is, and what other people think doesn't count. It's all about what I want." Giving up that bastion of identity is harder for many people than simply courteously servicing someone that you aren't into personally.

Q: We're both subs—should we switch off? Or find a dominant who will take both of us at once?

Raven: Ah, the double sub problem! I've seen it before. Generally the solutions tend to be either to switch off, or find someone to take you on as a couple, if only occasionally.

Ways I've seen the switch-off done: I know one couple who does it by six-month situations. Every six months one formally becomes the slave of the other, and then they switch six months later. The only thing was that they both had to vow that nothing done during the "submissive" period would be carried over into the "dominant" period—no petty vengeance for giving the other one a hard time. Other folk prefer to switch every other time, or something much more short-term like that. It's largely a question of how long each of you can stand to be dominant before the urge to be submissive overwhelms you— an hour, a week, a month?

I've certainly also seen people dominate—and own— couples, and I've topped couples myself. It can be a very good thing for a master/mistress who doesn't want to get involved with a falling-in-love thing with their subs or slaves, but wants those subs or slaves to have access to intimate emotional affection. The couple gets their service needs met by the dominant, but gets their emotional love-needs met by each other.

Questions you would need to ask yourselves, and have worked out before you find a dominant:

❖ Are you primarily interested in kinky sexual submission, or is this more about nonsexual lifestyle? Do your desires largely center around the sexual aspects of power and control (with SM thrown in), or does cleaning someone's house and humbly serving them in other nonsexual ways give you great emotional benefits? Do both of you answer those question the same way?

❖ The answers to #1 will help with #2: Are either/both of you actually looking for someone to own you as a couple, or would you prefer just a top who would periodically play with you, and only have (limited) authority during those times?

❖ Does the idea of living in someone else's space and being part of their "household" appeal to you, or do you want to live in your own space together and commute to your service?

❖ Are you both heterosexual, or not? Is the gender of a master/mistress important, or not?

❖ Most telling and difficult, if the two of you want to be owned as a couple, how much authority would you be willing to give to an owner regarding your relationship to each other? For example, what if an owner decreed what sort of sex you could have with each other, restricting certain things (orgasm? penetration?) only for Themselves? What if they demanded to know the intimate details of your relationship, or insisted on mediating your quarrels and demanding that you take their advice? If this sort of thing makes you flinch and say "Arrgh!" then you need to have clear limits set on how much interference a D/s relationship could have between you. (Obviously, you need to be very careful in finding a dominant who respects and approves of your relationship, and is invested in the two of you being together rather than attempting to break you up or cause trouble between you.)

Frankly, Joshua and I have often fantasized about getting other slaves for the house, and our agreement has always been that the perfect situation would be a slave couple, ideally both extremely bisexual masochists, hard-working, obedient and service-oriented. They'd be two extra obedient pairs of hands around the house and farm for the price of one, two extra incomes to add to the household, and they could tend to each other's whip-welts, kiss away each others' tears and lend emotional support after I've reduced them both to whimpering wrecks, have Joshua train them in tandem, and be family members of a M/s household, and neither would need to fall in love with me or my boy. Not to mention how much fun it would be to force them to do various perverted things to each other that they would never think to do on their own ...hmmm... Nice thought, although we'd need to add a wing to the house first!

Q: In households where there are multiple slaves, is there a hierarchy? If so, are the ones in the middle really switches?

Raven: While currently I only have the one slave, I've had more than one sub at a time in the past, and possibly will again, depending on circumstances. (It's not like you can go buy them at the Wal-Mart.) And yes, I tend to go with alpha-slave hierarchies. Obviously not all masters/mistresses do that. It would depend on the whims of the owner, and the character and abilities of the specific slaves.

My boy Joshua makes an excellent lieutenant, in the sense of being able to carry out my orders with regard to people underneath him. On his own, he doesn't have much leadership charisma or ability, but with a mandate from me he can "borrow" authority from my word, and keep folks in line. I've sent him to herd people (in non D/s contexts) for me short-term, and he can manage that. He doesn't always make judgments well enough to be the one on the top of the pyramid, but with someone above him to check his decisions he's fine. He's also a good trainer of submissives, and I can very much see him in a majordomo position. So if we got other slaves, he'd be the alpha.

As to the rest, I am in fair admiration of a multi-slave household that I once visited where the slave hierarchy was: Alpha slave (long-term partner) on top, then those who'd been there more than a year and committed to staying, ranked in order of their ability to manage others below them, then newcomers ranked in order of seniority. I thought that was pretty sensible.

I realize that some slaves are just unsuited for any kind of authority, and that others may need to be on a very short leash for reasons of judgment, but the average slave can certainly handle carrying out the Owner's orders by supervising other slaves in the matter. After all, anyone who holds a day job where they are higher than the absolute bottom worker has to do that.

Some households incorporate physical punishment and/or SM and/or sex into the hierarchy, making all but the lowest slaves into de facto sexual switches. Some keep the hierarchy only for doing work. I've done the latter, although not the former; I think it might be a good call for a household where you had a punishment context and a *lot* of subs of various sorts, and depending on the single owner for sex/SM/attention/etc. would guarantee that they didn't get much at all.

Actually, I'd think that the single biggest problem with a multi-slave household is the amount of the owner's time and attention that each slave would want, as opposed to how much the owner can actually manage to give them. At some point, the owner might find themselves entirely taken up with giving the slaves time and attention, which some might find to be great, but it seems that in some cases giving attention to one's slaves might end up being a full-time job. People often underestimate how much time a new relationship will take up in their life.

Q: Why don't you talk more about your wife and how she fits into all this? I'd like to hear more about the details of your poly dynamic.

Raven: Because she's asked me not to, and she guards her privacy, and out of respect for that I will not discuss her and our relationship any more than I have ... except to say that we have been together for 16 years and it still works. She's not the public person that I am (and that I require Joshua to be), and she has the right to remain private.

Community Customs

Q: Oh, come on. Master/slave couples aren't living in the real world.

Raven: To answer this question honestly and with regard to reality, I expect that M/s couples live to varying degrees in the "real world", depending on who we're talking about. To me, "living in the real world" doesn't mean "doing what everyone else is doing just because they're doing it". It means *taking the real world into account and modifying my behavior appropriately.* For example, I can't walk down Main Street with a string of naked slaves on a chain. We'd get arrested. So I won't. I'll have naked slaves at home, where there will be no legal repercussions and will not offend or horrify nonconsenting bystanders. That's living in the real world. I use what some people might consider conditioning techniques to get my slave to do what I want, not attempting to make the law force him to do that—because I see no evidence that it would. That's living in the real world. I don't tell my slave to do illegal activities just because I could. That's living in the real world.

The truth is that the "real world" often has little tolerance for any minority lifestyle. As a member of several minorities, that doesn't mean that I have to submit to that. It means that I have to be realistic about the obstacles between me and what I want for my life, and do what I can while not overly risking the safety of myself or those dependent on me, or my sense of ethics.

Having a M/s relationship has not gotten me arrested. It has not lost me my community, because I have handled it appropriately (meaning downplaying it sometimes, not discussing it sometimes, doing education sometimes), and because I made real-world decisions about where I chose to put my time and energies. It has not cost me respect from anyone whose respect I cared about. It's a matter of good judgment.

I think what people mean when they say "not living in the real world" is that a member of an unaccepted social minority will often create a small pocket of space where they can "live as if" those outside mores did not exist, by use of good boundaries that prevent outside authorities from interfering. As long as those boundaries are designed to buffer and not to blind, that's still very much taking the real world into account. Those people, like myself, are still very much aware of those social mores, and it may be a source of pain to them. If they actually believed that those mores did not exist, and acted that way, they'd probably be arrested. The fact that nearly all of us remain at large suggests to me that we do indeed know how to take the "real world" into account.

Of course, sometimes what is meant by "you don't live in the real world" is "You don't live in *my* world," meaning their internal worldview. And no, I don't. But I hope that I am aware enough of most people's own little worlds that I can communicate across that gap.

Q: Is M/s legal? Isn't there a way that the Law could get the owner for kidnapping, or coercion, or something?

Raven: I'd like to point out that legal repercussions for M/s depend entirely on the ability of the State to procure A) the s-type's cooperation in claiming that they were, indeed, coerced or made to do anything that they did not desire and actively seek, and/or B) evidence that the s-type is not mentally stable. If someone cannot be proven to be nuts, and they say, "Yes, I want that, I asked for that," then it's much harder for the State to apply those laws...

...except in places where the laws are set up by the State to ignore the existence of meaningful consent. By this I mean laws that are based on the idea that Activity X could not possibly be anything but harmful, and/or that no sane person could possibly agree to it willingly, and therefore by definition the activity is harmful and the people involved not sane or safe.

These are the laws where you can't consent to your own "assault", even if you were on your knees begging someone to whip you. People have already gone to prison for this.

Those laws are a whole different bowl of chips. They make a mockery of informed consent, and they are the basis for defense of "deprogramming"... of anything not currently socially acceptable. It's those attitudes and laws, in conjunction with otherwise reasonable anti-cult rulings, that scare me more than any cult.

Q: Why is the majority of the BDSM community, and even the D/s/M/s folks, against internal enslavement? Can't they just say that this is a risk-aware situation, just like anything else?

Raven: Because when you're dealing with a situation where someone cannot leave, and cannot disobey, whether or not it is safe is completely dependent on the morals, ethics, and sanity of the owner involved. Period. If they had the bad luck or bad judgment to pick a lousy owner and then get themselves psychologically enslaved, then they're fucked.

Internal enslavement has the potential for far, far greater damage than voluntary submission, if it's done badly. We *are* playing with fire. Some people *will* get burned. We need to respect that, because if we go about pretending it isn't so when it so obviously is, we will lose what credibility we have left.

Contrary to what some IE practitioners say, I don't believe that being a bad owner means that the slave becomes unenslaved. It is quite possible to internally enslave someone into total psychological submission and then do horrible things to them. Those techniques are available to unethical people as well as good ones. That's what the other people in the BDSM community are afraid of happening. It would be lying to say that it couldn't happen. All you can say is that it isn't happening *to you*, and try to give a counter-example. They will come to this with their own worries and fears.

People for whom the lack of agency and free will required to be a slave would be damaging are going to have a hard time imagining what it's like to be someone for whom that's a good thing. I know, because I'm one of those people. I make a really lousy slave, and it screws with me big time. For the longest time I couldn't understand the kind of psyche that would thrive in slavery, because it's so different from my own. I had to have it explained to me by thoughtful and articulate submissives before I could get my head around it. That's what we're up against, and I understand how horrifying it can look to someone for whom it isn't suitable.

Q: Do you ever do Daddy/boy or Daddy/girl play?

Raven: I can't do Daddy/girl. Partly because I raised a daughter, and it was not sexual at all for me and it feels weird to think of it that way. Partly because I'm not heterosexual enough to do that cultural dynamic—not that I can't be attracted to women, but I can't seem to manage the male-female social-role chemistry. I tend to treat girls like boys, which tends to confuse them utterly (except the ones who say, "Thank God! Someone I can be a boy with!") so I generally refrain.

On the other hand, I have done a good deal of Daddy/boy when I was working out my shit earlier on. I think that I worked out 90% of my abusive father issues playing that stuff, although I was never Daddy, I was Papa (with the accent on the second syllable) and my father persona was rather Victorian or debauched aristocratic. But for me the emotional heat was always in the same-sex dynamic there, the fact that I was slowly growing someone who'd been in my (theoretical) place to come to be where I was now. Which means that, by definition, the "boy" grows up and leaves.

In America, there are two different connotations to "boy/submissive male partner". One's ageplay. The other is the deliberate infantilization of adult men in service positions—

houseboy, etc. Once I'd worked out my shit, I found that I didn't want to do ageplay any more, I wanted a "service" boy. So I don't do ageplay with Joshua. He finds that whole thing creepy anyway.

When we first got together, he denied that he had any father issues, or if he did, that they were influencing his choices. He had a weak, erratic, and needy father who dropped out of his life around puberty, and a bunch of large thuggish immature violent uncles. He's admitted since then that his first boyfriend was (psychologically) him dating his father, and his second boyfriend was him dating his uncles. I seem to be like none of the men in his life growing up. I suppose, given their caliber, that's a good thing. I don't push the issue, because it still creeps him out, but I can't imagine that a boy with a history of poor male role models whose favorite sexual partner is a dominant older man *isn't* working something out there. I'm hoping that the message has been, "See, it doesn't have to be like that."

Q: Should all submissives defer socially to all dominants?

Raven: There are some private groups where one of the rules is just that—while you're there, if you're a submissive, you are expected to be at the least deferential to any dominant members. Private groups have the right to structure themselves any way that they like, and if you go there, you're implicitly consenting. However, I think you're talking about the average leather bar or BDSM munch or play party, or even general online forum.

My advice to submissives is to be polite but not submissive to any dominant in such venues with whom you do not have a negotiated power dynamic. Guard your boundaries, and politely inform anyone who attempts to trespass on them without your consent that this is not acceptable. If they persist, leave and get the host. If you know that you're the sort who has trouble keeping your boundaries solid, you might try making an agreement with a "mentor" dominant or more experienced submissive who will "chaperone" you. (This is assuming that you're free and unowned. If you're under the care of a dominant, well, it's their decision as to how to handle this.)

I advise this because in a public group, you cannot guarantee that all the self-proclaimed dominants in attendance are going to be experienced, courteous people who know how to respect boundaries. You have to protect yourself against the percentage who are the opposite of that. Simple politeness, on your part, is enough to show basic respect and show off your submission; you need not take orders from anyone who makes you uncomfortable.

Joshua: I can understand why someone might think all dominants should be treated with a higher than average level of respect ... if they believe that being a dominant is a notable achievement requiring skill, dedication, hard work, and so forth. However, if all that is required to "be a dominant" is to check off a box on a form and stick a title in front of your online name, it is ridiculous to claim that it is a status worthy of the respect of complete strangers. Claiming that someone, somewhere, obeys you and grants you the highest respect is simply not going to convince most people that you are anyone worth deferring to.

Even in real-time BDSM communities, with few exceptions, there are no qualifications whatsoever for being a dominant. By many people's standards, you don't even need to have (or ever have had) a submissive of any description to qualify. You only need to identify as dominant. Any position which can be bought this cheaply will not command the respect of a reasonably intelligent mixed group of strangers. In practice, of course, those who wish to demonstrate the depth of their submissiveness to the public will defer to all and sundry, and those who don't will generally refrain.

Q: What does "collar of consideration" mean?

Joshua: I've mostly heard it compared to being engaged to be married, but there seems to be a good deal less assurance of a permanent relationship coming of it than that would imply. Perhaps it is more like "going steady", sort of like giving a girl your class ring or pin.

In many cases it seems to be a matter officially marking the submissive as the (current) territory of the dominant. They've now got a big "No Poaching/No Trespassing" sign on them. Casual flirting/playing with this one is off limits, unless it goes through the dominant; if you treat this submissive in an inappropriate way, this dominant will likely have something to say about it. Local community standards really define what this entails, though.

I once knew a prominent woman in Philadelphia who would accept submissives under her "protection", which was in many ways treated like "consideration" (that is, "no trespassing without permission") without any implication of a current or potential sexual, romantic, or sadomasochistic relationship between herself and them. She mostly did this for newbies or women with a history (or fear) of making poor decisions about which men to trust. She would arrange occasional "safe" dates, and talk to potential partners to screen out the unrepentantly sleazy.

Q: We are married and have children, but we want to work toward M/s. How can we do our M/s dynamic in front of them, without letting them know about it?

Raven: It seems that what you're is asking is whether there can be a strict protocol that does not give attendant children any idea that there is D/s going on. Yes, there can be, if both parties are honest and imaginative and have good communication, and are more interested in discipline for its own sake rather than something sexually titillating. We don't have any kids around any more (grown and flown!), but we have a whole lot of vanilla people who don't want to see or know about the M/s part of our relationship. We happen to live with some of these people, and interact frequently with others. Add to this the fact that we have many houseguests, our back field is a retreat center in the summer/fall, we have church events here on a monthly basis or more, and I *cannot* be seen by clueless people treating someone in a way that could be read as abusive or disrespectful of their boundaries.

This means that our dynamic needs to be very, very subtle. It's a matter of working out a "code" that looks normal, and no one has to know that it stands for underlying D/s orders. We act vanilla in public, and have verbal codes between us that only we understand. For example: We are in a kitchen full of church guests. I want him to fetch me a drink. He has been having a conversation with someone, and they don't notice that he subtly steers them into a place where he can keep an eye on me and I won't have to look for him.

I say, "Sweetie, will you fetch me a drink, please?" He knows that I mean "Get me a drink, boy. You know what I like." He says, "Sure, hon." I know that he means Yes, sir. He smiles and fetches the drink for me, being careful not to look inconvenienced in any way. If he looked like he was less than completely happy to "do this little favor for his partner", it would make me look bad. I say, "Thank you, love." He knows that it means "Good boy." Yes, we're playacting for the benefit of the onlookers and their comfort, but it's playacting that is discussed and mandated, and he's doing it on my orders.

As another example: if we are at church choir practice, and someone needs a ride to pick up their car from the mechanic down the street, and I feel like pimping my boy out to do that, I'll say, "Hey, Josh, would you be OK with taking Joe here down the road?" Because we've worked it out first, Joshua knows that this is Egalitarian Mask for "Josh, get the car and drive this guy, and act like you are happy to do it even if you hate the idea, and tell him it's no trouble." His response is, "Sure, that'd be no trouble," with a smile, even if he's cringing because he hates Joe or really doesn't want to get up again and run an errand. Joe would likely be uncomfortable if he knew that A) to what extent Josh is my slave, and B) that he didn't have a choice in the matter, and that discomfort would make difficult my sharing of resources in order to help someone. So nobody has to know.

In public, where people can see it, he is to appear for all practical purposes to be my eager-to-please partner, my "perfect boyfriend" who just happens to always want to do what I want to do, who is amiable and charming and a good sport, and obviously loves me. Who is clearly intelligent and independent of thought, enough so that he can't possibly be a brainwashed doormat, he must be fetching and carrying for me because he honestly wants to, because we're a team. (The fact that I'm a crip helps. When I've got the cane, people don't wonder why he's carrying the luggage.) This means that there are even specific (minor) areas that he's allowed to disagree with me on in public conversations (cheerfully and respectfully), because it adds to the fiction for the onlookers. Do we enjoy this? Not always. Sometimes it sucks, for both of us, but we don't live in a fantasy world.

You might pick a specific endearment for your dominant—like "sweetie" or "beloved"—and declare that when you say it, you're really saying Sir. When he says it back to you, or perhaps says another endearment, it means "That's an Order." Perhaps a certain kind of touch can be understood code for "I'm reminding you that I own you," or the like.

Since what you're doing is hiding things from your children—a difficult thing that will work only so-so at best—it will involve implicit or explicit orders to be acting or faking it for their benefit. That's life; it's that or wait until they are grown. But that acting will extend to both of you. Your master should be able to make a polite request in a mild tone with Please and Thank Yous—setting good examples for the kids—and you can mentally "write in" the commanding voice you'd rather he be using. You can reply in a way that is cheerful but not submissive, and implies that you're acquiescing because you love him and are happy to help—also good examples for the kids—and he can "write in" the implicit "If it pleases you, Sir." Talking this all through beforehand can help.

My point is that even when people are around and you have to act vanilla, there are ways to make that about service as well. If *you two* know what's really being said, that's what's important.

Q: You're both very public about what you do. Are there any communities that you're part of which disapprove, or give you a hard time?

Raven: Most would, actually. We are active in a number of communities, and most of them have no clue about M/s, and would find it discomfiting. This means that we have to be careful in those places to behave in ways that take the focus off of that part of our relationship. If people asked, we'd discuss it privately with them for educational purposes, but we don't bring it up, or act in ways that would make people think of it when we're there.

For example, I have a leadership role in my church. Our religion is completely fine with GLBT relationships, and polyamory. The demographic makeup of our church is about 25-30% nonheterosexual, and there are quite a few poly folks. BDSM is a different issue. Some are tolerant of it (and the core group/Church Council is fine with it), but the majority are fairly uncomfortable, because it resembles abuse superficially on the surface. I'd say that the majority could be made OK with S/M, but D/s—and specifically M/s—makes a lot of people uncomfortable. It is too difficult for people to understand that this is not a violation of someone's rights, and especially that the internal enslavement we practice is not just a form of evil brainwashing that I am visiting on a helpless person ... in other words, that there's no difference between Joshua and some woman suffering from battered woman's syndrome.

I think, also, that a lot of folks are very sensitized to authority figures who look as if they are abusing their authority, or that they *might* do so ... especially women. As a male authority figure in my church, I have found that (non-submissive) women are extremely skittish around me if they see me treating my partner in a nonegalitarian manner. The issue of abuse is too close for them, and it smacks of cult-leader megalomania to them. ("If he treats someone he *loves* this way, what's he going to demand of me eventually? What, does he think he's David Koresh?")

Even some of the people who know about the situation—and I should point out that we are not closeted, I give workshops on spiritual BDSM to my religious community and I've written the only book that I know of on the subject of doing it in my religious context—are sometimes uncomfortable when they see it happen in public, because it triggers their issues. That's why it's important that I appear to be someone who is extremely invested in respecting the rights of other people. Which I am! But saying that won't help. Modeling it is what helps. That means playing down things that people find triggering. (It helps that my wife is obviously such a non-submissive individual that I couldn't possibly be a tyrannical cult leader and be married to her.)

There are other things I don't do in that community. I don't flirt, with anyone. I don't act in a sexual or even sexually aware manner with anyone (my partners excluded), and I don't project sexual energy. I don't treat anyone as if I expect them to hold to traditional gender roles. I go to a great deal of trouble to project "Safe", because it works. It's made things much easier; I'm much more trusted. (You have to understand that four women so far, all basically strangers to me, have walked up and informed me that I remind them of their abuser for some strange reason they couldn't figure out which, they admitted, had nothing to do with my behavior. Being an alpha is very threatening to many people, even on a subconscious level. Men, too, but they usually just try to start fights with me, and that's easier to defuse and handle, assuming no one is drunk.)

It's a line that I've chosen to draw. I would not belong to a church that felt that way about GLBT or polyamory, because that's about the very existence of my lovers in my life, and the legitimacy of our being together at all. I wouldn't be in a church where I couldn't hug Joshua in public and call him Sweetie. But the M/s line is a much more controversial, and it would be nigh impossible to find a group of people who are good with all the other stuff that the folks in my church are great about, and were entirely cool with M/s, and were in my area! It's a sacrifice I'm willing to make.

And meanwhile, I'm putting my money where my mouth is, and educating, educating, educating in my religious community. Maybe in 20 years things will have changed. I believe that I can manifest change if I try hard enough, but it won't happen quickly or without my hard work. So rather than bitching and moaning, I'm creating change.

Q: My friends claim to be egalitarian, but they're always having power struggles, and one of them is completely henpecked. But they would never admit that this is D/s! Is it, really?

Joshua: To me, deception like this is the most destructive thing. A big reason that I *like* small-scale hierarchical social structures is that the power is aboveboard. Everyone knows who is in charge and the people in charge are held accountable. Ideally, anyway.

Cue my *Rant of an Angry Servant*:

In "egalitarian" social forms, the power is so often just as unequally distributed as in an overtly hierarchical arrangement, but when things go wrong, I've all too often seen the folks who really have the power step back and claim that as they are all "equals"; "everyone" shares responsibility for the problem. That too often ends up with everyone else actually shouldering the burden for the bad decisions and poor leadership of those who are covertly in charge, getting none of the benefits of power and all the responsibilities. The people in power cannot be called out for their mistreatment of those under them, because no one will admit that anyone has power over anyone else. Claiming that your inferiors are actually your "equals"—and insisting that they do the same—does nothing to level out a power imbalance and everything to hide accountability.

Speed Bumps and Smooth Sailing:
When You Know You're Doing It For Real

Practical Issues

Q: If you own a slave, do you own their money and possessions as well? How does that work?

Raven: As usual, that's something negotiated in the beginning, and it will be different for everyone. But I certainly do. If I own him, I own everything that he owns. That includes his money, and his things. On the other hand, it means that I am responsible for making decisions about his clothing, schoolbooks, and other things that he needs.

I didn't intend that in the beginning, because I have a lot of intense issues about money myself. I'm very possessive about my money and my things, and it was difficult for me to relate to someone who was happy to hand it all over and let someone else make decisions about it. I was also iffy about taking someone's savings away before I knew if this relationship was really going to live up to its advertising, so what I told him was, "I choose to have you steward it responsibly for me until such time as I decide to do anything with it. Ditto your possessions." A year later, I fully took charge of it. We opened a joint account, and while he has access to it, he needs my permission to do anything other than pay the bills I've ordered him to deal with.

Joshua: When I took up with my master, I made it clear to him that my all financial resources and everything I owned was entirely at his disposal. Of course, at the time my financial resources were pretty much limited to a credit card with a $2000 debt, a trunk of clothes, a small crate of books, and an old laptop. I suspect my winter coat and boots were the most valuable items. I may have had a little bit of cash, but not much.

I had thought it was a little silly when my master initially declined to have any involvement with my finances. At the time he brushed it off with comments like, "What do I want with your credit card debt?" Years later, he told me that part of the reason was that until he was really sure this was going to be a permanent situation, he did not want to feel an obligation to get me financially back on my feet if he dismissed me. I was to remain just as able to support myself as I was when I came to him. When he finally determined that I was appropriate for the position and was able to commit to him for life, he took control over my finances. Certainly, I wouldn't mind having no assets in my name. I don't mind having them either. I don't feel like I have any more control over them just because they are legally mine.

At this point I work part time and provide most of my master's financial support. I added his name to my credit card, because I have good credit and he has almost none, and my credit is also a resource for him to use. I've got a debit card for a joint account where my paycheck is deposited and he doesn't have to worry about giving me money for gas and groceries. He takes money out of the account as he pleases and I only spend it as authorized. I used to get explicit permission for every purchase, but now there are a number of things that I know I can just buy while I'm out if we need them and let him know afterwards. (Toilet paper, soap, certain foods, gas, etc.) He has his own account as well, but he spends from my account as he likes. I am responsible for seeing that our bills are paid on time, and I have standing orders about what I may purchase on this account without prior approval. To be fair to the other folks in the house, bills are split evenly among all of us. My master is responsible for making sure both my share and his get paid, but generally he does that by having a standing order that I pay both shares out of my account. He is not a spendthrift and makes good decisions about where the money goes, and I trust him with overseeing our financial situation.

He's never expressed concern over me having "unsupervised" access to money. He sends me to do most of the shopping, so it is convenient. Even when he comes shopping with me, he often leaves to sit in the car before we check out because he doesn't want to stand in line with his arthritic joints. Also, my master may be thrifty, but I am downright cheap. He's quite confident that by my nature I would never spend money on things he found frivolous. In fact, he's chastised me for not buying myself lunch when I've been out all day. (I say, "But it is too expensive. I should have brought something." He says, "But you didn't. You need to eat.")

If I were to be dismissed from service, my master would have no obligation to see to my financial support. I'm an adult, and capable of looking after my own needs. I would turn over the entirety of my bank account to him before leaving, and he would settle up any debt he had in my name.

Just as a historical note ... apparently it used to be that liveried male servants did not own their livery. It wasn't unheard of for surly male servants to be threatened with the forcible removal of their livery if they tried to storm off.

Q: What's the hardest thing about not owning your own money and property?

Joshua: There are two things that it is sometimes difficult for me to not own:

First, pocket change. I was in the habit of giving change to homeless folks, kids raising money for Little League, the Salvation Army bell-ringers, and all manner of people. My master only approves of giving change to street musicians. (He used to be one.) This is sometimes uncomfortable for me.

Second, food. We've got five adults in our household. Because we all eat very differently and have a limited food budget, we don't share most of our groceries with each other. So I can get a little proprietary over "my" muffins, or "my" leftover Chinese. When I find that while I was at school my master has eaten both my leftover Chinese and his own, I might be a little grumpy. It is his right, of course, but it is one of those things that reminds me that I don't actually own anything. Not even half a pint of cold lo mein. Nothing.

Not owning my car, or house, or clothing, doesn't matter to me one bit. Not owning canned peaches does.

Q: If you own the slave's money, do you own their debt as well?

Raven: Yes. You do. Once they're enslaved, you can keep them from running up more debt, but if they come to you with debt in hand, it's yours just like they are. You can set them to paying it off—we know of one master who made his slave work in a fast-food joint for months and turn over all the money to pay off pre-existing debts—but you've got to decide before taking them on whether this is something you're willing to deal with.

When Joshua came to live with me, he had a few boxes and bags of books and clothing, a few bucks in his pocket, and $2000 or so in credit card debt run up from medical expenses and not having insurance. I paid it with my next book royalty check, which came many months later, after he was committed to me. The debt payment happened right after the official ... well, I won't call it collaring because we don't use a collar. Enslavement ceremony, if you will, which was really more of a formality because he was already quite enslaved by then. So it marked me officially taking over all his finances and property. It kind of felt like I'd made the slave-auction payment and "bought" him, in a way. It sealed the deal, as it were. Sure, it would have been nice if he came without debt, but it was a small price to pay.

Q: Should a master move in with a slave, or is that just Not Done? Does it have to be that the slave comes to the master's house? For that matter, shouldn't the dominant support the slave financially?

Raven: I'm one of those masters whose slave supports them. While I didn't move into his house—I already owned the house, so he moved into mine—I'm semi-disabled and I'm probably never going to make more than the tiny pittance that I already do. He's able-bodied and skilled, and getting more skilled all the time.

A slave is a resource for their owner to use. How they use them depends on what the owner wants. For me, a slave with a high-paying job (not that Josh has a high-paying job, but if, say, he was a lawyer or something) would be a useful resource that would be wasted by making them quit and be a house slave. (Unless they desperately wanted to quit and be a house slave.)

If my circumstances were different when we'd first met—if I'd wanted to live in a city, if I'd had no family and was open to moving, if he had a place that I liked—I could definitely see moving in on him, and basically taking over the place. Once he was owned, his house would just become an extension of my property. If you're afraid to let a slave have money or possessions (including a house) because they might use it without your permission and guidance, they aren't fully enslaved. If they're fully enslaved, it's all just an extension of your stuff.

When it comes to models of dominance, the overriding social one that we all grew up with (if only in the ever-present media) is that of the heterosexual male breadwinner whose power and authority comes in large part from the fact that he provides for his dependents. This role has permeated most people to such an extent that it winds its way into people's ideas of how dominants should and should not act, regardless of their gender and other factors. We need to shake the idea of the 1950s father-knows-best dominant—the (putatively male) dom works the job and the (putatively female) slave stays home and is a traditional housewife, just in chains—as the Only True Way to do a power exchange.

Female dommes with male subs are in a particularly sticky place with this, because men often have more chances for better income than women. As such, it's perfectly acceptable to see a sub with a better job than you'll ever get as a resource to be utilized. A submissive can learn to feel useful to someone by supporting them financially. I know a few married submissive men with traditional wives who didn't know that their husband secretly wanted to be submissive; and while they wouldn't have approved, the men decided to "see" going to work at shit jobs every day and faithfully bringing home a paycheck to support their wives as submissive service that they were offering. In essence, they mentally cast themselves as paycheck slaves for the women that they loved and cared for, and this helped to carry them through the drudgery of every day.

I'd like to point out that throughout history, the people in dominant positions at the top of society were not the ones who went out and labored every day. Your average medieval lord didn't go out and toil in the dirt—he had serfs to do it for him, and turn over the fruits of the work to him, and he supervised how things were to go in his demesne. Was that "mooching", or was that tribute, a fair exchange for a fair exchange? (And lest you think that no one today would want to be a serf, remember that most people would think that no one today would want to be a slave, either.) The lord's job was to manage things, make the far-reaching decisions, and put himself in harm's way should it come to protection. (In a modern context, when the cops or the tax man comes to the door, it's the dominant who handles it.) This is the model that I use in reframing the fact that I'm not the breadwinner. I don't need to be.

Most modern consensual "slaves" fall into a continuum of wanting control vs. wanting to be of service, an issue which is described in our section on service and control. I've noticed that the control-oriented ones often tend to want to stay home and not work a job, and encourage the idea that the ideal owner is a well-off breadwinner. The ones on the service end tend to be fine with working and supporting the owner, because it's a form of service. Heterosexual female submissives may have the worst time with this idea, because it's all too easy for them to romanticize traditional straight gender roles as part of their M/s, and become resentful when they aren't fully supported and are expected to work and contribute, perhaps because their dominant isn't wealthy enough for their fantasies.

Actually, speaking of money, that's another meme from bad BDSM porn that I'd like to expunge—the idea that dominants are supposed to be wealthy, and that money is one of the measures of how dominant someone is. The corollary to that is the idea that wealthy people have the right to demand respect and submission just because they're rich, regardless of what sort of reprehensible idiots they might be. That's a flaw in many otherwise intelligent and creative BDSM novels, where the only real criteria for being a slave-owner is a large bank account.

Q: Does the owner have the right to choose or change a slave's career? Even an established one?

Raven: When I met Joshua, he was getting a degree in computer programming, but he was also deciding that he didn't want to work in an office-type job, so it was easy to have him abandon the degree and come live with me. (Before everyone flinches, please understand that we discussed this thoroughly, and decided that there was no point in him wasting any more time on a degree for a field he wasn't going to enjoy.) Yes, the money might have been better, but if I was going to be in charge of making decisions about his future career, I wanted it to be one that he would enjoy, and that would be flexible enough time-wise as to not interfere with regular service to me. Ideally, it would be a service to me in ways other than a mere paycheck as well.

I decided, after he'd been around for a couple of years and I knew him and his talents and proclivities, that he would be damn good as a massage therapist. That career fit the above standard, and it meant that I would have a live-in on-call massage therapist as well. So I arranged for his education, and sent him off to it. Luckily, I guessed right—clients have been continually saying to him, "You're certainly in the right job!" Since then, he's gone on to get a degree in complementary health care, and training in acupressure Shiatsu, Asian bodywork, and traditional Chinese medicine. These extensions of his career were ones that he came up with, and I approved. It showed that I'd chosen well, and that this field would be a good one for him, for talent and interest both.

My point is that while the owner does indeed have the right to choose the career for the slave ... well, I hate the idea of waste. There's a balance to be had between the owner's convenience and outright wasting some talents and abilities. A slave is a resource to be exploited in the most effective way. Using every slave as a hammer when you've actually got a scalpel, or a screwdriver, or a chamois dust mop, is poor leadership. (I'm not saying that the owner doesn't have the right to waste the slave, assuming that they agreed to that in the beginning. I own my car, and I have the right to total it, or never drive it. But that'd be damn stupid of me. Just because you *can* do something doesn't mean that you *should*.)

If you go changing their career to suit yourself, make sure that you know very well what kind of tool you have in your hand before you go assigning it a toolbox. Make sure that you are not blinded by some idea about what sort of tool they *ought* to be. You might want to get outside help—a career counselor who could help them find a similar career with fewer hours and less commitment, maybe? Someone in that field who's "downgraded", perhaps due to having kids, and could give advice? And if you decide that they have to quit entirely, perhaps having them give volunteer work with those skills? Joshua still does computer stuff—he maintains my website and formats my books and is an all-around pet-geek on call. Waste not, want not. Remember that word: Resource.

Slave Health And Owner Health

Q: If a master/mistress has an occasional meltdown, or sick day, where they are in no shape to make decisions, what should they do about their slave? Will the slave lose trust in them, or be frightened, if the master/mistress is not able to be in control of them at that moment?

Raven: I think that it depends on the slave. Some slaves really need their dominant to be a rock all the time. (Probably bad for the dominant psychologically, but hey, not my call.) Some (often more "caretaking" sorts) are fine with intense displays of emotion ... so long as it doesn't interfere with the dominant's ability to function, and function better than average, in daily life. The same goes for sick days, or any other time that outside circumstances leave the dominant unable to function well for a short time.

I've got a chronic illness that sometimes leaves me a physical wreck. Sometimes the pain and sickness is bad enough that it leaves me an emotional wreck too. I'm tough, but no matter how tough you are, there's something that can wear you down and break you, at least for the moment. The reason that Joshua is fine with this is that:

❖ he would rather have honesty and intimacy than a false facade of perfect stoicism;

❖ he has instructions as to what to do when I'm in that state (how and whether to comfort me, what will help, what protocol to follow, etc.) so it's not an uncertain situation for him;

❖ he knows that I am skilled at gauging when my judgment is somewhat off and I need to not make important decisions during that time (like, say, when my blood sugar is terribly low) and can admit that without an issue;

❖ he knows, from experience, that I will pull myself together in reasonable time and get back in the saddle, and it doesn't affect my ability to handle things for any significant period of time.

As long as those things are true, he's fine with me occasionally being a wreck. I think that's true for any reasonably secure, sane, and service-oriented sub. What makes for trouble is when either the sub has so many psychological insecurity issues that they can't interact with a fully human dominant, or the dominant doesn't take the sub's need for protocols in emotionally uncertain situations into account, or the dominant is allowing breakdowns to affect their decisions. If a sub is having a problem with their dominant's bad days, coming up with a specific list of things for them to do/say/act when it happens will help. Making sure that bad days don't overwhelm the dominant to the point of affecting their judgment is useful too—could they do what I call a "left-brain override" in an emergency and pull it together if necessary?

Of course, this requires that the owner have a strong enough ego to be able to admit that there will be days when they really aren't up to hands-on slave management. You can't make protocols for a situation that you aren't willing to admit exists.

Q: Obviously, an owner should be responsible for a slave's health, because they own their bodies. But what do folks think about the ethics of making decisions for your slave that are arguably not optimal to their health, but well within the normal range of behavior one could reasonable expect a person to engage in? (I'm not talking about the master's *right* to do so, but the ethical issues s/he might consider in making the choice.)

Joshua: Those are difficult decisions. For instance, consider a slave who desires to be thinner and when left to their own devices will diet strenuously. Perhaps their master likes them at their current body weight—even if they are on the plump side. Perhaps their fixation on dieting is annoying to the master, or a distraction from things the master finds more important. Perhaps the master doesn't care for having diet foods around the house or for his/her money being spent on them. Perhaps the master likes going out for cheeseburgers or ice cream occasionally and would like a dining companion. It may not be optimal nutrition, but it is fair enough.

Or to use a personal example: I am allergic to cats. My master's daughter had two cats for some years after I moved in. It didn't kill me, but it certainly wasn't optimal to my health. I've lived with housemates who had cats in the past, because the rent was cheap, but obviously I'd be healthier if I didn't. He did not judge my allergy to substantially limit my usefulness, but it did get me wheezy and sniffly occasionally. If he were to put maintaining an environment optimal to my health and well-being as a high priority, this would be a problem. Instead, he had a looser standard of "healthy enough", and the level of allergen exposure falls in that range. The cats are gone now, as his daughter has grown up and moved away with them, but there's still dust and mildew. However, he's not going to buy a new house just so I won't ever sniffle.

To be clear, we're not talking here about asking a slave to start smoking crack or having rampant unsafe sex—nothing that could be considered reckless endangerment. I suppose the issue is: what level of health does the master feel obligated to maintain in a slave? The practical answer would probably be: A level of health equal or better to the level that they maintain in themselves.

There is a range of behavior between willfully or recklessly damaging, and ideal optimal care. If you own a vintage Rolls Royce, you are likely to come quite close to optimal care. If you are a busy single mother with a 10-year-old minivan, you aren't going to go whacking it with a 2x4, but you also may not get the oil changed as frequently as you ought to, and you will likely not buy premium components or repair every ding and scratch. Or perhaps I just like to think that I can withstand a good amount of wear-and-tear, and not be much worse off for it!

Q: What about when the slave is sick? Does the owner take care of them? If an owner tells the slave to stop serving them and putting them first until they're better, does that mean that the relationship has to be egalitarian for a while?

Joshua: My master does a certain amount of taking care of me when I'm sick, and definitely looks out for my health and wellbeing. He doesn't generally fuss over me or go wildly out of his way for me, but he will give me extra physical affection when I'm sick and he might bring me a bowl of soup or something.

Early in our relationship I was under the impression that it was best to just go about business as usual. I was running a high fever one day, and after doing an astoundingly poor job of washing dishes, my master not only sent me to bed, but told me quite firmly that if I am sick I am to let him know immediately. Sometimes work will need to get done whether I am sick or not, but I need to give him the information so he can make that decision.

I think the best thing he's ever done was to order me to go to the doctor for a long-term problem when I had been trying to tough it out. He's occasionally ordered me to do certain things to maintain or improve my health, but on the whole I'm expected to maintain reasonably good health without assistance, make healthy lifestyle choices, etc. It's part of safeguarding his property.

Raven: It's quite possible to take care of someone in a dominant way. Every parent does it for their kids. Do you think that you know what's best for your submissive? Of course you do, or you wouldn't be telling them that they aren't to serve you until you decide they're well. Has it occurred to you that this is still you deciding what happens? (One hopes.)

Let me put this a different way. Being in charge means that you decide how the interaction is going to go, and the slave goes along with it. That can be, "On your knees, wench!" It can be, "Honey, I'm tired. Take care of me. You know what to do." It can be, "Do the dishes and then get me a beer." It can be, "You're running a fever, put the dishes down and go to bed already!" You decide when it changes from one to another.

In the Owner's chapter, I discussed different styles of mastery. I tend very much to the "celebrity" end most of the time, but when Joshua is ill or hasn't done his homework or is trying to do something that is bad for him, you want to see how fast I snap into a parental style? It's a matter of what the situation warrants. A dominant saying, "You're sick, stop serving me and go to bed," is just a matter of changing styles.

Q: Can an owner have their slave be their personal trainer? Can they be enlisted in helping the owner to be healthy? How is this accomplished without nagging?

Raven: Absolutely they can. I had my boy learn tai ch'i so that he could train and coach me in it. He is supposed to make me healthy food to eat, and encourage me to eat it. He gets to remind me to do things, but it doesn't create a problem in the dynamic, because we both know that I could say No at any point, and there would be nothing that he could do about it. He is expected to take the No gracefully, and not nag further on any given day.

If there's a problem, it's because he honestly wants to keep me healthier, and it's hard for him when I do say No and use the Owner Override. But that's a matter of him keeping things in perspective. It's his job to be an aid for me in these things, not to make me do them, and he has learned not to take it personally. The slave needs to remember that dominants tend to be stubborn individuals, and nagging generally achieves the opposite effect of what is intended. The slave also has to remember that it's not their business whether the owner exercises today or not.

And if what you need is a personal coach/cheerleader, why not? After all, isn't the slave's job to make the owner's life easier? Just remember that it's completely up to the owner to set the attitude with which the slave is to do these things for them. They can order it to be done in a way that doesn't push their buttons, or make them feel resentful and unwilling to do the work. As with so many things, the owner has to keep in mind that if they don't like the slave's behavior, words, or attitude, and they have the right and the ability to change it, then they should do so. However, as a corollary, they also need to be self-aware enough to be able to figure out where their own buttons are, if they want to keep them from getting pushed.

Q: I want to keep my master healthy. But he can tell me to fuck off while he does unhealthy things, and I can't stop him. What do I do?

Joshua: I know that my master hates to take care of his health, and hates the restrictions that physical disability puts on him. Part of my job is to be his nurse and caretaker. I try like crazy to be supportive without nagging. I can attempt to make healthier choices more appealing and convenient, but that's really all I can do. It is entirely his choice.

The biggest issue with his health is taking it easy when he's having a bad day. If he doesn't, he gets sicker ... and sometimes, he gets sicker for no apparent reason and then "taking it easy" means a few days of bedrest. I am afraid I do nag him terribly about this, and am frequently out of line on it.

From a service perspective, it is difficult dealing with how much he hates to ask me to do things for him that he can't do for himself. He has no trouble asking me to do things he could do, if he chose to, but to *need* my help is really hard for him. So many personal services are hugely emotionally weighted for him, because where another person would see the service as a luxury, he sees it as the mark of an invalid. I have to find that line between expressing eager willingness to help and acting as if he can't be expected to do it himself.

It is intensely frustrating. When I'm in a bad mood, all I can think is, "What kind of lazy-assed boy do you think I am?" and "I didn't give up my whole friggin' life so you could then spare me the inconvenience of doing my job!" At the same time, I *feel* like a lazy-assed boy for not doing every bit of housework that he could possibly decide to attempt while I'm away at work. I feel like, "If only I had washed all the dishes, and done the laundry, and this and that, maybe he would have taken a nap this afternoon," and "If I worked harder, then he wouldn't waste his time on stuff that I *can* do, when he has a hundred more important tasks that I *can't* do and limited energy to do them with."

There's no really perfect answer. At best, perhaps you can talk to him about how much you depend on them, and how scared you get when they don't take care of themselves ... but make sure that you do it in a way that is clean of anything that could look like manipulation. In the end, you have to trust them.

Q: Sometimes I ask my owner what I should fix for dinner, and I get the answer: Food. Is this supposed to be dominant and decisive?

Raven: I do this. Basically, there are times when I don't want to have to decide what to eat (when hypoglycemic, for example, when all food looks lousy but I must eat or die, or when I'm in the middle of obsessively working). Joshua has been trained in what to do at that point. Instead of asking what I would like to eat, he brings me a list of choices (not based on what would be easiest for him to fix, either—we had to set that limit—but based on what I've trained him with regard to my preferences and health) and lists them to me. If I am still not interested in deciding, he makes me something healthy that he knows I like and puts it in front of me, and I eat it because at that point I barely care.

I don't see how that's so much of a problem, as long as the servant has been briefed with what the master/mistress likes, and what acceptable choices would be. Perhaps you could phrase your question like this: "Ma'am, I'd been thinking of making glazed chicken for dinner, or possibly reheating the eggplant casserole that needs to get eaten up. Would either of those be preferable to you, or is there something else that you'd prefer instead?" That leaves her the option of making a decision or not, as she chooses. Sometimes it can be a great luxury to not have to make a decision and be guaranteed it will come out in a way you like anyway. Remember that. After all, a slave is a luxury service.

Joshua: A submissive once mentioned that their master says, "It's not *my* job to figure out what I want," when faced with these situations.

Q: How do you keep your owner from feeling down and depressed during illness?

Joshua: Oral sex. Really good oral sex.

Okay, seriously, sex is no panacea, but my master has a tendency to hate and resent his "broken" body, and good sex really seems to help him feel like it isn't all bad. Sometimes he hurts too much and is too miserable for any kind of sex, but he usually still enjoys being touched and cuddled and massaged. Touch is very important.

Also I try to always keep in mind that while my master occasionally does things that exacerbate his condition, no amount of healthy lifestyle choices are going to make him entirely well. The amount of clean living he already does quite faithfully is substantial. As he's gotten more careful about his health, I've also come to realize that his remaining "unhealthy" choices serve a vital role in maintaining his emotional well-being. I know he chafes under the restrictions that his illness places on him, and at my best I do what I can to ease that burden rather than pushing for further restriction.

For instance, he's very allergic to certain food dyes, mostly reds and blues. Aside from the obvious assistance in checking that his food is safe for him to eat, I try to find foods he normally wouldn't be able to eat that are actually safe. Bright red pastries often cheer him up—the "all natural" ones that are made just with berries or are dyed with beet juice extract. I even found a bright red "natural" soda pop last week. I've occasionally sorted the "poisonous" colors out of M&Ms and removed colored frosting from cupcakes. It's all part of my continual mindfulness in trying to make him happy.

Aside from indulgent snacks, I do try (as much as I'm able, with work and all) to make him healthy food that he actually enjoys. For him this means as much organic food as we can afford or produce ourselves, and very little processed convenience food. It means leaving wholesome food in the fridge when I'm at work—at best, ready-to-eat plates that only need a few minutes microwaving, if that. I don't make "diet" food, but farm food with simple ingredients. He really likes good, wholesome food, and he loves food that just magically appears when he wants it. I've encouraged him in exercise when practical, but his health comes in cycles.

For a while, I think my master needed some assurance that I would not leave him because of his illness, and I would not see him as pathetic or undominant because of it. He is by now quite confident in my loyalty and obedience to him, and he's even coming to accept that I find him intensely sexually desirable in any physical condition. I suppose that brings us back to the therapeutic value of enthusiastic oral sex, eh?

Q: Can a disabled person own a slave? If so, what should they expect of them?

Raven: If you're disabled and you acquire a slave, it's probable that you'll end up having them be your PCA (personal care attendant) as time goes on. If you don't have one yet, being your PCA is one of the things you need to put on the list of Must Be OK With. In terms of training, there are a lot of organizations that train people to be PCAs. If you're getting on disability pay, check with the local bureaucracy for such resources. There are many family members, for instance, who end up being caretakers for their parents or spouses, and need some training for this, and there are organizations that do that.

Having a slave to train as your PCA is a wonderful thing. There's no embarrassment around them helping you with bodily functions like there would be with a hired stranger, and a good slave will find a way to make you feel like this is a luxury service, not just something done because you're in a bad way and can't do it yourself. You can figure out what sort of (non-medical) care you might need, and send them to learn how to do it. They can bring you your medications, they can cook you special food, they can carry things for you, they can clean your house, they can give you sexual services.

This assumes, of course, for a special breed of submissive. Being a disabled dominant is a drawback to finding the right submissive, no question. You do need a slave who is a natural caretaker, and who is very service-oriented. All too often I run across submissives who require that their dominant be healthy and able to physically overpower them in order to feel properly "slavey", not to mention never having days when their master is too debilitated by pain to cope with "acting" dominant.

My boy Joshua has written something in an essay that I will quote here:

> *...In most BDSM porn, if there is a notion of a worthy master, it is often based on their ability to maintain control through constant displays of strength or superiority. I've heard folks in D/s relationships discuss what ought to be done if the master becomes ill and can no longer keep his slave "in line". This is entirely*

contrary to my idea of service. In this life, you provide service in times of strength and of weakness. You are serving a fallible, human master. If you cannot care for your master after his stroke, push his wheelchair, and consider him no less your master, you have utterly failed him and failed yourself.

And yes, for the record, you can top publicly from a wheelchair. And it can be impressive, especially if you tie the bottom's hands to the chair arms and drag them about on their knees while you beat them, occasionally shoving them up against the wall with the wheels ... and the bottoms in question know that you aren't going to take any whiny shit from them about how much this hurts.

In terms of sex or SM in general, it's the submissive's job to get themselves into whatever position is necessary in order for you to do what you need to do. If I'm in too much of a bad way to get up and fuck my boy actively, he can damn well get his ass to wherever I can reach without getting up. They're supposed to make themselves available, and part of that is making it easy for you to do it. Remember that. As the dominant, you need to make it clear that it's their job to be a "helpful victim", as it were.

Q: What about a slave with disabilities, or a slave who's usually healthy but has an accident or a long period of illness? How can they continue to serve?

Raven: I've spoken to quite a few submissives who struggle with illness and/or disability, and even the healthiest can fall off their bike and end up in traction for months. For the particularly service-oriented ones who are used to actively *working*, this can be very painful. They may believe themselves useless if they're too crippled to do their jobs, and their self-esteem may suffer. It's adding insult to injury if they're bad enough off that their dominant has to wait on them while they are laid up.

How well they cope will have a lot to do with their dominant's attitude. If this is a temporary situation, the dominant can keep refocusing them on getting better—eating properly, taking their medication, exercising, sleeping enough. Even if the focus for the submissive has largely been service, it can be switched to control, and their greatest service can be doing their best to get better by submitting fully to the process.

If the problem is an ongoing disability that isn't going to go away, the submissive needs to carefully choose a dominant who understands and is fine with that set of limitations. Instead of dwelling on what one can't do, concentrate on what can be done. Some control-oriented masters don't require that their slaves labor, only that they be charming and attentive and as obedient as possible. Some will confidently step into the role of health coach and create a regime to help their slave keep what health they have, and compensate for the rest. Some simply want human "pets". It's all a matter of finding the right one.

I am reminded of the submissive whose joints were too decrepit for her to kneel before her master, so they found another stance for her—bowing while holding out her hands—to show her submission to him. Another mistress had a slave who was wheelchair-bound; she did push his chair in stores, but he held the packages and was "parked" to wait in long shopping lines for her while she wandered about looking at sales. Even a slave who can't type on a computer can take care of annoying phone calls to the cleaners and the electric company. It's all a matter of patience and imagination.

Q: What happens if my dominant dies or the relationship ends? Won't I be bereft? Is it worth it?

Raven: It's a very good point, and one which should definitely be considered. We've discussed this a lot, since my boy is 14 years younger than I am, and my illness will likely eventually do me in. Our decision was more custom-tailored for him—he is very drawn to monasticism, although he's neither Catholic nor Buddhist. There's a part of him that very much wants to be an ascetic and live in spiritual community, in a monastery. That part of him had to be put aside in order to be with me. We decided that the best thing for him to do—because he doesn't want another owner, for reasons personal to him—was to go into a monastery when I'm gone. Since our particular religious denomination has no monasteries at the moment, this means that I have to start (and fund) one before I go. It will be my final gift to him, for all his years of service, and it will make sure that he has a place to be where the quiet spiritual discipline that he loves will be an everyday thing.

I've known other owners who made deals with other dominants that they trusted; if they die or go mad, the slave is transferred to this other person. While this is hard for someone who was in love with their owner, it's assumed that the slave will be deeply in mourning for a long time, and this at least gives a transition that does not have to push them back onto their own two feet during their grieving period. For slaves for whom service comes well before love, this is a good option, but it means that the owner needs to have enough friends who are decent people to have a trusted friend to give them to.

And as for not wanting to submit if it might end ... Everything ends. That's like saying that you don't ever want to fall in love and commit to someone because they might get hit by a bus tomorrow. Life doesn't work like that. All relationships are inherently risky. If you never risk, you never gain anything worth having. Calculate the risk, yes—but unless your prospective owner has a terminal disease that will do them in by next year, assume that everyone is going to die eventually and this is no excuse for putting off what you want from your life. (And even if the latter tragedy is the case, it still might be worth it.)

If you have a full-time submissive and you are pretty sure that it will be temporary—that they were going to be with you for while and then move on—ideally you'd still feel somewhat responsible. A good plan would probably be to have a cache of money, perhaps a CD or other account, that you could hand over as part of their release. Perhaps a part of any money earned during their time with me would be put aside for that time. Also, make sure that they have a career that they could pick up again (assuming that they'd put it down for you, which wouldn't necessarily have to be the case), and if this required getting them preparatory training, well, training in anything makes any slave more useful and valuable.

In terms of the psychological, you could have someone(s) designated to take care of them for a while, people that they could move in with who would buffer things for them. Perhaps a sort of "mom" or "dad" or "big brother or sister" to be with while they got their feet under them; someone you trust, someone who would have an existing relationship with them, if only platonic and respected.

It might be important for a slave to get over a master before taking up with another one, especially if they were dead. All sorts of idealization could happen then; they might forget about the fact that the late master was a human being with a large intestine and liver and sinus cavities, etc., and give a future dominant a very hard time for not being them. That's not fair to the next owner. They need to get the last one out of their system first before they can cleanly approach another D/s relationship.

If they dump you for another dominant and go straight into that dominant's house, without any negotiation, just sprung on you—which is what happened once to me—then of course they get nothing.

Obstacles

Q: I've been chronically depressed for the past year. It's made it very hard for me to obey my owner. What can I do?

Raven: I don't have any advice for you as to what will help your depression, because that's a very personal thing for you to have to work out on your own. However, I do have advice for your owner, and for every owner: If you own human property, and they have an illness that they came with, you are going to have to manage not only them but their illness. You should learn everything you can about their illness, from them and from outside sources. You need to be the one who consults medical personnel and makes sure that they are getting the right treatments, going to their appointments, taking their meds, avoiding irritants, etc. You're in a position to do this, and it's your job anyway. If you can't take responsibility for their health, you should release them to someone who can.

I have seen an awful lot of dominants who, when they find out that their sub has a physical issue that will get in the way of convenient service, don't want to know or hear about it. They want the sub to take care of it and keep it out of their sight, and this is wrong. It's like not wanting to think about your car ever needing oil. Sooner or later it will bite you in the ass.

For a mental illness, this goes twice as strongly. If your submissive has an uncontrolled mental illness, the illness is in control of them, not you. They will need some kind of treatment, as soon as possible. While not every mental illness is treatable, you owe it to them to try to get them the best help that you can. You'll also find that training and behavior modification slows to a crawl and doesn't "take" well during a period of chemical depression. I've noticed that while my "Jedi mind tricks" don't work on a chemically depressed (or, I would assume, otherwise chemically impaired) slave, once the chemical problem was alleviated, all the orders that I'd put in suddenly came through and worked. It was as if they were stuck in the in-box, as it were.

It's not an easy thing. I know one woman who had to sadly uncollar her submissive because the mental illness issues were just too big to get around, even with treatment; there were still too many outbursts and too little ability to obey. There aren't any miracle cures, and you can't dominate someone out of a chemical imbalance. A dominant can help a lot with things like personality disorders and trauma-induced psychological problems, but only if they are experienced, very knowledgeable about mental health, very committed, and otherwise really know what they are doing. If the latter qualities are not dead certain, they can do more harm than good.

It's not easy to find therapists who are comfortable with a power dynamic. You might look at Kink-Aware Professionals to find one, but even if you can't and you must hide the real nature of your relationship, most good therapists ought to be fine with you as their partner being involved with their treatment, and coming to arranged meetings with them and your partner. They might also appreciate careful notes from you about how new medications are affecting your partner, and most will appreciate your commitment to helping them get better, and a statement by your partner that "My partner is the person who I've made a promise to, a promise that I won't harm myself, and they will hold me to that in any way they can."

Q: Sometimes I go off the deep end, and yell at my master. It's low blood sugar, and something I can't control. How can I start to get a grip on this?

Joshua: I'll give you the benefit of the doubt and assume that you're already doing everything in your power to regulate your blood sugar. We'll assume you're having this problem despite appropriate medical care, healthy well-timed meals, and exercise. Obviously those are all things that you (and your master) can control, and should be controlling.

So given that, it is useful if you can manage to insert some comment about your mental/physical state when you go off. "I hate you, I hate you, I hate you! I'm hysterical, and I have low blood sugar, and I hate you." I've found that a good master is generally unmoved by hysterical outbursts, and will address it as a behavioral problem, rather then getting drawn into it and getting angry or upset about it.

If your master knows you have a blood sugar issue, he might be able to respond to the first signs of hysterics by asking about your blood sugar. The question might get you angry and defensive for a while, because in the moment you may feel like your emotions are entirely justified and have *nothing* to do with what you had for breakfast, but in my experience you get used to it. Being aware of what you are doing, in the moment, is the second step in getting the behavior under control. (First step is sincerely believing that you really are doing something that you'd rather not be doing.)

Third step (in my book) is being able to modify—in however small a way—the way you expres
s these emotions. That is about moving from 100% out of control to only 95% out of control, getting your foot in the door. Apply some protocol or restriction to your hysterical behavior. Nothing big! Nothing with huge emotional impact. For me, that step was not swearing at my master. I could yell at him, but no swearing.

Another technique is to ask permission to get hysterical, so long as he is willing to grant it. (If he just says no all the time, right off, you'll likely do it anyway and feel doubly bad about it.) Once that behavior is ingrained, he can put a short delay in. "We'll talk about this upstairs." And so forth. Even taking a few small steps like this can go a long way to convincing yourself that you *can* keep this behavior under control. The goal isn't that you never express these emotions, but that you learn to express them in an appropriate way, in an appropriate time and place. Of course, keeping your blood sugar regular will make things so much easier.

As a mindfulness tool, my master bought me this little pocket alarm, and it is amazingly useful. I can set it to vibrate every 5 or 10 or 15 minutes, and it reminds me to pause and do a little assessment of where I am at and what I'm doing. I can ask myself, "What are you doing right now?" If the answer is, "Pacing back and forth in the kitchen, thinking about how much I hate _____" then I can ask myself, "Is this what I want to be doing right now?" Every once in a while, I decide that, yes, brooding is exactly what I want to be doing right now, but in another five or ten minutes I'm going to have to answer that question again. And again. It makes it much harder to build up a good head of steam against anything.

Q: You've talked about the slave being the one to change, and the master helping them to do that ... but what about when the road to change is blocked with barbed wire, erected in childhood? How do you get past that?

Raven: Oh, I so wish that I had a clear or easy answer for you.

All I can say is that the two of you have to fight through that barbed wire together ... and that, unfortunately, the owner has to get to a certain point of both skill in the process and knowledge of the slave's psyche in order to be a good partner in this. Just being supportive is not enough.

I'm also a believer in desensitization, slow erosion over time of that barbed wire. You go up to the wire, you push a little, you back off. You clean up the mess. Then you do it again, as soon as you can bear it. And again, and again. A little further each time, and eventually one wears through, and wears it down, and then it has no power. The owner's job is to make the risky decision as to what's too much, and what's not enough. Likely they'll make mistakes. I have. You clean up the mess and try again. The hardest part is making the slave do it again after you've erred in judgment over too fast vs. too slow.

The thing to remember is that if there's really no way down that road, there's no wire barrier. The road just ends. The wire barrier means that there is a road, you just have to get through to it.

Q: What about slaves with neurological problems, like ADHD or autism?

Raven: My boy Joshua has a mild care of Aspergers Syndrome, and some comorbid brain dysfunction, so he has fairly serious memory problems, both short-term and long-term. He can't remember much of his own childhood and adolescence, although he can remember being able to remember it … the line of poor memory just keeps moving forward. We've compensated by having him use written lists and check them off and I do check up on him regularly. As he mentioned earlier in this chapter, we got him a little pocket alarm which can be set to go off in ten minutes, or to go off on a regular basis to make him aware of the time and shake his brain out of whatever posthole it's fallen into. (I have many times discovered him staring off into space, having become mesmerized by a wall pattern and entirely lost the last ten minutes.) We call it the "Josh, where's your brain?" timer.

The first thing was to figure out through trial and error what he could not reliably be trusted to remember. For him, this was about three simple verbal instructions at a time, less if he's in a loud and overstimulating environment. This is the first step—figure out your slave's neurological limits. Do this with an attitude of neutrally finding out what limits you have to work with; don't let it be about how quickly they'll fail you, or anything negative like that. You can deliberately set them up to fail at something as long as you then tell them that it was just a calibration test and don't make a big deal out of it.

Joshua functions much worse in high-stimulation situations—such as serving at a noisy party or following me around and being my attache when I'm presenting at a busy conference. Although I personally dislike formal protocol, these are situations in which the formal protocol is very necessary for him to function up to par—he needs to know exactly how to act and what to do, down to the smallest thing, so that he can concentrate on that.

Since these are public non-BDSM events where showing our power dynamic is problematic, we've worked out a protocol that does not draw attention to him and is more like that of a formal servant. He is not required to make small talk (which flusters him terribly in high-stimulation settings) and refers everyone to me; he is trained in how to be "in waiting", and so on. And, sometimes, he needs to go stand in a quiet place for a few minutes and collect himself before his brain starts screaming. He is trained to let me know when he needs this, before it gets to the bolting-out-of-the-room phase.

Aspergers Syndrome, in general, is characterized by a love of order and sameness, keeping down stimulation and the need to adapt to new things. Being a submissive or slave under strict discipline can be very comfortable for such a person, if they also have a submissive personality. Knowing exactly what is expected of them every time makes them feel very safe. I've also known Aspergers dominants who use enslavement as a way to have a partner who they can depend on to help uphold their neat, quiet, rigid life preferences

As an example of training difficulties, when the dominant tells an Aspergers sub to do something and they miss it, they may be being overstimulated and are shutting down input to cope. If the dominant makes eye contact and talks in a loud voice, that may be distracting. Having the sub close their eyes to listen to them, or telling the sub things in a specific quiet monotone might help. Aspergers people have trouble picking up on subtle social cues, which the dominant may be using to impart information and not understanding why the submissive doesn't get it.

Another classic Aspergers trait is the focusing on one detail. "Get me a glass of water." Aspie sub wanders out to

Mantra

kitchen, sees that no glasses are available, comes back in, says, "Will a mug do?" Most people would have made that mental leap, but he's stuck on "glass". That means that there will be a lot of rules that will seem self-evident, but that aren't, and will have to be created as people go along. "When I ask for a drink, these are the acceptable containers to bring it in, regardless of what word I use." And like that, depending on how bad the Aspergers is.

ADD and ADHD are different, in that they are often characterized by impulsivity and mental scattering. This is the opposite of a knack for order and discipline, but conversely an ADD sub who fully submits to the process can be helped by a patient and well-organized dominant who is willing to crack down on them. ADD disorders share with autistic-spectrum disorders a difficulty with screening out excess stimuli, especially in loud and varied environments. For example, to keep the submissive focused during play, you might give them a short, simple verbal mantra to say.

If you want the submissive both to pay attention and to actually learn something, you will need to provide a *very* quiet and unstimulating environment. I say this from the perspective of a parent with an ADHD child who was bad enough that she had to be homeschooled. What we did with her, if we actually wanted her to absorb and keep something mentally, is to work with her in a quiet room with *no noise*—and that means no background music, no cars going by outside, no neighbors or housemates banging around, no phone ringing—and low visual stimulation—boring walls, etc. She did best with only one other person, one-on-one, and when that person kept some kind of light, grounding physical contact with her, like a hand on her shoulder. No stroking—that's distracting stimuli, not grounding stimuli.

Understand that overstimulation (like painplay while distracting a submissive with talking) can cause neural overload and a freakout. It's not emotional, it's the brain-wiring screaming. A good way to calm ADHD people down is to hold eye contact, holding their face if necessary, and do a breathing exercise with them. (We did that with my daughter when she would get overstimulated and freak out as a child; we called it "the wind game". But don't do it with an Aspie—eye contact makes freakouts worse for them.) This means that if you see the submissive freaking out, the first thing you need to ask is whether they're overstimulated and need to sit down, close their eyes, and breathe.

In terms of the memory issue, which is a problem for both ADD-types and autistic-spectrum types, writing things down helps. Lists, lists, lists. My boy makes lists, I hand him lists, I have him type out lists of rules to look at. Don't just make lists of things to do, make lists to remind you what order to look at your lists in. ADD types may need a lot of checking up, at first, to make sure that they haven't wandered off. Here's another area where a beeping timer can help, giving them a signal to refocus on their task.

Some neurologists claim that you can't have autistic-spectrum disorders like Aspergers at the same time as ADD or ADHD, but that's nonsense. I know of at least two Aspergers people (not my slave) who also have ADD. Aspergers is not medicable, but the other two are ... sometimes. Medications can help, or they might not. They always have side effects, some of them negative. They work better for some people than for others. If a dominant takes on the responsibility of ordering their slave to get medicated for ADD, they need to make sure of these things:

❖ That they are not going into it with a "this will fix my slave" attitude—they need to be able to comfortably let go of it as a solution if it seems to be not working, or not working out.

❖ That they are willing to learn a great deal about the various ADD medications, and who they work best for, and their side effects,

❖ That they are willing to talk to the submissive's doctors, and take their advice, and get them to explain what they're giving and why,

❖ If medications work, get a med-minder to remind them to take the darn things.

Basically, it's a matter of figuring out what their limits are, and working within them. The less you can make the submissive feel bad about their disability, the better.

For those that use a punishment dynamic: don't ever punish them for actions resulting from the neurological disorder. It's totally unfair, as it is not "curable" and only somewhat compensatable, and it is totally unhelpful. I don't care how much a dominant thinks that everything is built of people's beliefs and is subject to change. No amount of training, discipline, or love is going to make a neurological disorder go away. It's not going to happen. It's as if the submissive came to the dominant on crutches and was punished for not being able to walk. That's not the way it works. They need to accept the fact that the slave comes with a disability, and go from there.

In order to work with this disability and learn to compensate for parts of it, the dominant needs to know everything about it. They need to devour information about it, especially material for parents helping children to cope; they might even think about talking to parents of kids with these disorders. While these are (assumedly) intelligent adults, the information carries over, especially for someone who is training them, and creating an atmosphere that the submissive will be forced into. The dominant needs to accept the limits of the submissive's physical brain, and how much can or cannot be done.

For submissives with these problems: Please, please do not sign up with a dominant who is not living in reality about your condition. That's like a car owner who refuses to believe that cars need oil and brake fluid and transmission fluid as well as gasoline. If you own a slave, you need to learn everything about how they work, and there will be some things you can't change and need to work around. Thinking otherwise is hubris. I can't stress that enough.

Joshua: I think that Aspergers makes my service both harder and easier, but it makes everything in my life both harder and easier. It is easier because I don't naturally have a really firm sense of how "normal" interpersonal relationships are supposed to go, so any reasonable and internally consistent model of relating to people makes as much sense to me as any other. Talking to other autistic-spectrum folks, we seem to have an easy time adapting to radically different relationship structures. We tend not to internalize social rules very well, and if we're emotionally invested in a set of social rules it is usually more an aversion to learning new rules when we already had what seemed to be a perfectly good set ... but with unusual ways of relating, people are much more likely to explicitly discuss the roles and rules and expectations. No one does that in normal "dating" or normal social situations. Being given a clear rulebook is so nice.

I have no trouble with all manner of "arbitrary" rules for my behavior, because my natural perception of society is that we all live under tons of arbitrary rules of behavior, with varying degrees of social enforcement for them. As children, there are all sorts of things that autistic-spectrum people do, and have to be told not to do, that it would never occur to a "normal" to do. *Don't chew your clothes. Don't sniff people when you are introduced. Don't wave your arms around like that.* These seem at least as arbitrary to me as any M/s rules, and a good dominant will actually put effort into *training* you in the M/s rules.

Raven doesn't often do strict formal protocol, but I love it when he does, because the stricter the protocol is, the easier it is for me to relate to people. What "normal" people see as a casual social situation with no rules for behavior seems to me like a minefield of unspoken rules that they all find agreeable.

The strict protocol is wonderful because you learn a comparatively small number of behaviors and the exact rules about when and where to apply them. That sounds sort of "robotic", but that is really comfortable for me. In fact, the formal protocol is a lot of what drew me to D/s in the first place—not because I find it sexy, but because it is so comfortable. Acting "normal" and "natural" doesn't feel normal or comfortable at all. It is like doing hour after hour of improv acting when you have no way of telling if you're doing it well. With formal protocol I know exactly how well I am doing, and I love that.

The Aspergers does make me fairly literally minded; sometimes I'll get tripped up over which things are actual meaningful qualifiers on an order and which are just the way it happened to be phrased. I've mostly learned to tell the difference, but for example I still routinely get tripped up on being asked to do something "quick". Does that mean instantly, or as soon as I'm done with this? At a faster than usual pace, or at a normal pace but no dallying? Or does it only mean the person making the request is feeling harried or wants to emphasize that they are not imposing on me with a time-consuming request, in which case it does not apply any meaningful modification to the request at all?

Raven is really patient with me on this, and while he won't go out of his way to make his requests 100% unambiguous, he will clarify when I ask. He might give me the Look (the "my boy is so strange" look), but I know he doesn't think less of me for it. Aspergers also makes it easier and harder because Raven and I have a very emotionally intimate relationship, and I'm often very emotionally insensitive. There are a lot of things I don't realize are hurtful. I've learned a lot about that and I am much better, but it is still very difficult. Certain areas of my emotional development were very delayed. I came into Raven's service at 22, and my relationship skills were closer to 12. I was very mature in some ways, but I think Raven was a little shocked to see how uneven my emotional development was. He was willing to do a lot of "motoring through" with relationship skills (and he was very good at it), and I don't know that things would have worked out otherwise.

On the flip side, being emotionally insensitive means that I take criticism very well. I don't get hurt or offended, because it doesn't usually occur to me to attach any emotional importance to it. If Raven is in a bad mood and is short with me, I don't take it personally. I've learned by rote how to identify "grumpy" behaviors, but I don't instinctively react emotionally to them, so it is easy for me to internally define certain behaviors as "Raven in a bad mood" rather than "Raven thinks I suck".

Another difficulty is that my service to Raven often involves being charming and being in very stimulating social situations. Thankfully this is usually only weekend conferences—I would really struggle with being "on" in that way on a daily basis. But sometimes I do ask to run off and hide in the pantry during loud parties because it is just too much.

Sex In A Deep Power Dynamic

Q: Should a slave be allowed to complain about not getting orgasms? Since when do they get orgasms?

Raven: When it's important to their owner that they do so. Certainly, a slave is not entitled to an orgasm. But if their owner says, "I want you to come," then they'd better get to it, if it's at all possible for them, whether they want to or not.

There are a variety of reasons why a master might want a slave to come. Perhaps they like the feeling of power in "making" them come. Perhaps they like it for ego purposes. Perhaps they think that the slave is fetching while moaning in ecstasy. Perhaps they like the contractions around their cock. Perhaps they are retraining the slave's sexual responses and learning to orgasm from new things is part of that training. Perhaps they like to feel generous and merciful and see the slave be humbly grateful for the chance to come. Perhaps they like the energy of another person's orgasm and like to feed on it. There are plenty of reasons.

I've certainly been in situations where the orgasm wasn't a reward. I played occasionally with one woman who finds it very easy to orgasm multiple times from a lot of different stimuli. I made her make herself come again and again and again, until she was tired of it and begs to be allowed to stop, but nope, gotta keep going at least three more times, honey. It's pure sadism, turning pleasure into pain.

Joshua came to me with a lot of orgasmic difficulty, and I insisted on teaching his body to come quicker and easier even when it brought up serious emotions and he was crying and sobbing after each come. To him, orgasm was vulnerability, and he felt safer and more reserved and closed-off when he was just being used without any thought for his own pleasure. Of course, I couldn't have that, not for a moment. Once it was easier and less complicated for him, once he'd come to expect it from sex, that was the time to start teasing and frustrating and denying it. More bang for your buck that way.

Q: What about restricting orgasms? When is that good and when is it a problem?

Raven: That depends on the sexual nature of the specific submissive. People are all different, affected by different hormones, early experiences, and relationships with their bodies. In some submissives it's something that you may have to discover via trial and error. In the beginning of my relationship with Joshua, we experimented with chastity and I discovered that not masturbating was entirely too easy for him. All he did was turn off his sexuality and disconnect himself from the neck down; it took him about two weeks to shut down entirely. Since he has a history of dissociation, it was nothing for him. Of course, this made it hard for him to turn it back on when I wanted him to be sexual. He also had a habit of using masturbation as a tool for general comfort, going to sleep at night, and (especially) waking up in the morning, and not being able to do that was frustrating to him, and not in a good way.

Since I have a busy life, and sometimes I don't get around to having sex for a week or more, this was a problem. The solution that we hit on is that he can masturbate all he likes ... he just can't come. This is adequate for the purposes of getting awake in the mornings, staying in touch with his sexual parts, and generally getting his energy moving, but still allows me to have complete control over his orgasms, which is a powerful thing for both of us. I also decided that if he was going to jerk off, he should work on how long he can keep himself aroused without coming, especially if he can stay right on the edge for a long time. It's very Tantric in its own way.

This has had excellent side effects beyond just the clear feeling of control and ownership. Being able to jerk off but not come is great for inducing sexual frustration, which I find delicious in a submissive. This relationship is the first one in which he's ever experienced real sexual frustration; due to his ability to easily shut down sexually, it never worked before. He got to experience for the first time begging desperately to come ... and really meaning it, really wanting it that bad. Also, his ability to control his arousal and orgasm patterns is improving. He has more of a hair-trigger now, and we're working toward him being able to come from new stimuli.

Chastity in a submissive is something that requires careful study of the submissive's sexual responses in order to be effective. Of course, there's the question of "effective for what?" For many dominants, the submissive's chastity is there to titillate the dominant, to make them feel like they are in control, and they don't give a rat's ass how it's working for the submissive—in which case "effective" is easy. For others, the idea is to keep them in a state of vague sexual frustration, so that every time their crotch throbs they remember how much they are not in control. If their crotch just stops throbbing— and it can, with submissives who have low sex drives, or sexual damage from earlier trauma, or are on antidepressants that lower libido, or are just really good at dissociating—then it's not effective.

I also know a few femme-dommes who use chastity on male bottoms in order to drive home the "it's not all about you and your hard-on" thing. Some of them go so far as to try and train in a "your erection is pushy and therefore unsubmissive and bad, so you won't have any" headspace. There are so many male bottoms out there for whom all this really is about their hard-on that I can see the appeal of doing things that way.

For the record, while we're talking about penis-bearing subs in general, keeping them without any ability to orgasm (for example, in a chastity harness that prevents erections and wet dreams even at night) for months and months is bad for the prostate. The prostate needs to empty itself on a regular basis or the prostatic fluid will build up and solidify, which basically means that it becomes clogged with toothpaste-like residue and can get infected, and in worst cases need surgical removal. Wet dreams are the body's built-in mechanism for prostate health, something which some owners (especially ones who don't have prostates of their own) may not understand.

Some femme-dommes have found that a good solution to this problem is to anally massage the sub's prostate about every two weeks, pressing the fluid out through the penis. If they don't want any erections or orgasms associated with the process, they can have the sub soak their bits in cold water until they are numb. This keeps the prostate healthy, is a pretty submissive-feeling activity (being ass-up while your Mistress gets the rubber gloves and clinically does the process "for your own good"), and can facilitate permanent chastity without too many ill effects. Of course, penises do shrink and wither a bit with years of disuse (I've seen this happen) and testosterone levels also fall, possibly causing testicle shrinkage. But it's reversible and not life-threatening, whereas prostate infections are Bad.

As far as I have read medically, women have none of these problems. But women are far more likely to dissociate from their genitals and their sexuality given prolonged chastity, and may be harder to "bring back" from that. Frankly, I think that regular orgasms are good for people, because they are a release of built-up negative energy in the body. Of course, "regular" can mean once a week or once a month, depending on the sub. In order to be really psychologically effective for a sub, the dominant needs to really understand the sub's sexual psychology, and not simply apply a one-size-fits-few fetishy rule because that's the way subs react in BDSM porn.

Q: All the BDSM erotica is full of slaves who can have hundreds of orgasms on command, but I have trouble having even one, especially with someone else present! I'm very service-oriented, and I always focus on the other person's pleasure at the expense of my own. I have a new master and I'm afraid that he's going to want me to have lots of orgasms. What do I do?

Raven: First, is there something creating the dissociation history? Gender dysphoria? Abuse history? Religious/spiritual issues? If so, that's going to have to be addressed first. If it's a cause that the dominant has no experience in dealing with (like an abuse history for a dominant with no experience with that, or gender dysphoria for a nontrans dominant), they're going to be stuck with fumbling in the dark. Not a fun place to be; I've had that happen with subs who had mental illnesses that I wasn't familiar with, and some things I just had to Leave Alone rather than make worse. Some things are jobs for Specialists. (I don't necessarily mean mental health people, although that could be the case. I mean people with experience in that area.)

Second, how important is it to your master that you be regularly orgasmic? How does that fit into his training plan? Is he used to subs who are constantly hard and turned on, and orgasm control gives him a leash via their cock to make them behave? Does he just like to be able to make his subs come easily because it's fun and powerful? Is he taking this on to help you for your own good? At the very least you should know how important it is to him. It may not be.

Joshua: Since you specified the problem occurs when you are with someone, I'm going to assume you don't have trouble reaching orgasm alone. I'm also going to assume that your master is interested in fixing this problem.

A really useful technique is gradually bringing your master into your private masturbation. Can you imagine him being there in the room with you when you jerk off—not with him being inside your fantasy, but as if he was right there watching you jerk off? Can you jerk off while he's in the next room, knowing he knows what you are doing? Can you do it without worrying that he'll hear you or walk in on you? Can you take pictures or video of yourself doing things while staying in your "private masturbation" headspace (not your "service oriented" headspace) and then show them to him? Can you jerk off while he's in another part of the room, within sight and earshot, but totally engrossed in some other activity and not paying attention to you? What if he's watching you? You might get stuck at the point where you are able to masturbate to orgasm with your master present, but not with him actively participating. A good in-between step is to have him to order you around while you are masturbating—having you stop and start, use different toys, whatever. That can help you to learn to surrender control of the overall experience while keeping the details of the physical sensations under your control. (And it is fun!) Keep increasing his involvement, until you can get yourself off during sex play with him in exactly the ways you do in private masturbation.

Once you've got that, you can work on increasing the variety of ways you can get off, but the goal here is to have a 99% success rate before you move on. That way, no matter what activities you are doing, you will always have this method as a "Plan B" if you are struggling to reach orgasm and he wants you to. Let me tell you, it is much more satisfying (for both people) to be able to switch to an effective Plan B then it is to give up entirely.

If you want this technique to work, it is very important that you not change what you usually do in order to make it more pleasing to your master, unless he specifically tells you to. If you start having trouble getting to orgasm, back up to a scenario where you can get off easily. Don't rush it!

(Okay, I'm sure you'll rush it no matter what I say, because you want to be the best boy possible as quickly as possible, preferably yesterday. I totally appreciate this impulse, but be mindful of it and be brutally honest with your master about where you are at, so he can keep you from rushing it. Let him set the pace. It'll probably be painfully slow, and you'll think, "I can do more than this! Let me prove it to you!" but he won't let you, and he'll be right. That's why he's in charge.)

The most important prerequisite for me was being with a partner who I knew accepted me entirely and would not reject me if I revealed every strange and unflattering thing about myself. I needed someone who I wanted to be emotionally intimate with, and who I trusted enough to "let go" in that way.

I needed to really accept and understand that my master thoroughly enjoyed giving me pleasure, in part because it was an expression of his control over my body and my mind. At first I managed to accept this only a tiny bit, just enough to make some progress on the issue. It was years later that I really understood my master well enough to understand this on a deep level.

I needed to understand that sometimes he cares whether I'm enjoying it, and sometimes he doesn't. When he really wants me to enjoy it, and I can't manage to, he is disappointed, but only a little. He is an adult. He doesn't expect to always get 100% of everything he wants exactly when he wants it. I needed to know I wouldn't be rejected or punished for letting him know I wasn't enjoying something. I needed to accept that I wasn't perfect, and that was okay. (Oh boy, is this hard! I still struggle with this.)

I needed to get over my silly idea that I masturbate "wrong". I'm actually embarrassed at how hard this was for me, and I still wrestle with it if my master wants to play publicly.

In any case, once I could really accept that receiving pleasure was a service, things got so much easier. It was really hard for me to accept that! Even though he told me it was so, I fought like crazy against the idea. But he won eventually, and he was right.

Q: What about female subs who use sex to manipulate their male doms? Should you put them in chastity?

Raven: You could ... unless the female in question is used to manipulating through flirtatious behavior, rather than actually putting out. Chastity won't stop that. The only thing that will stop it is the master proving that he can shut off all visible response to her physical attractiveness, at least for a period of time. The only way to take away that power is to make it repeatedly and clearly useless.

A gay trainer-dom friend of mine has been sought after many times by owners of female submissives who were having trouble being broken out of their habit of attempting to manipulate anything male (including their master) through flirtatious behavior. Generally he wouldn't let them know that he was gay at first, he'd just train them nonsexually for a while and totally ignore their attempts to flirt with him. When they were good and frustrated, he'd have them give him a blowjob, which he'd stop in the middle and critique, and tell them all the ways in which it could be improved, and then call out his slaveboy to demonstrate how to do it right.

At this point they were generally stunned, crushed, and feeling humiliated and uncertain. Then he'd say to them, "You see that you have no power here. You have absolutely nothing to offer me except your obedience. Now we can actually begin."

Joshua: If this is a persistent problem in a serious D/s relationship, I think that some training is in order. The submissive should understand that seduction is a power she has, and one that she must be willing to surrender. I would have her spend at least a month being as un-sexy as possible. This could include chastity, but not if she's the type to get sexually frustrated. You don't want her sexually on edge. You want her to find out who she is when she isn't being sexy. It might be more effective to have fairly mundane sex, or to be entirely indifferent to whether or not she masturbates.

These are the sort of rules I'd have:

❖ No sexy clothes. Boring underwear, utilitarian bras, flannel nightgowns. If she tries hard to stay thin, the clothes should be as bulky as the weather will allow. The goal isn't for her to look especially ugly, just plain and unremarkable.

❖ No makeup. No perfume or scented bath products. No hair-care products. No shaving anything. Depending on the situation, I probably wouldn't let her shower as often as she'd like to.

❖ If she has particular sexy mannerisms, they need to stop. I'd probably smack her whenever she did them, but ignoring her might work just as well.

❖ If she flirts with other men, she should have as little contact with men as possible, or only with men who will be entirely indifferent to her. When she settles in, it might be beneficial for her to have supervised contact with men who previously would have been seducible, but are not likely to notice her now.

I think it is very important to give the submissive the opportunity to excel in other areas during this time. You don't want her to feel worthless, and while she's sure to find it humiliating at first, the point is for her to get over that. Many women base their self-esteem on their attractiveness, and she needs to know that she is a good and valuable person even if no one wants to have sex with her.

Q: Should the slave be spontaneous in showing sexual desire? What if the dominant wants them to be sexually "forward" and show hunger? What if the dominant also doesn't like spontaneity?

Raven: I think it's perfectly OK to say, "This is the spectrum of what's acceptable, and you can do anything within that spectrum." It's a good middle ground between micromanagement and no direction. I do feel that in most things, my boy has pretty good judgment, and ought to be allowed to use it. Also, he has shown himself quite skilled at watching me and extrapolating what sorts of things I would like and dislike. (With some help from me pointing things out.)

So based on that, he's allowed a certain amount of freedom and spontaneity within certain boundaries.

For an example that compares sex to food: Sometimes I'm busy working, glued to the computer, and I just want some lunch. I don't want to think about what we have in the pantry, or even what I might want. I tell him to fix me some lunch, and he takes what we have on hand and comes up with something that he knows I'll like to eat, within all my dietary restrictions plus my need for variety. So one could say that it's spontaneous, but it can't be *too* spontaneous—"Uh...what the hell is this green stuff, Josh?"

And yes, I do like him to show desire and hunger in wanting me sexually. It's nice to be wanted, and to have someone who will show it, even if I don't always have the time to take them up on it that minute. (Actually, it's even nicer to have someone who will show it and then not be all hurt and disappointed because you don't drop everything and sweep them off to the bedroom for their efforts.) And it's fine for that to be spontaneous ... as long as it isn't done in public, or when I'm in the middle of some creative process that he knows I'll be irritated to be distracted from.

Q: My dom wants me to find being fucked sexy, and I don't. I was a virgin when we met, and only lesbian porn turns me on. How do I give him this? How do I throw off my fantasies?

Raven: You can't "throw off" attraction to women, or to any gender. That trick never works. If you were bisexual before, you'll be bisexual forever, at least internally. You can choose not to act on that, of course, for the rest of your life if possible, but those feelings are not going to leave you, and repressing something that big might cause a problem eventually.

But to directly address the main issue: The problem, from your post, seems to be not merely that you can't achieve orgasm during penis-in-vagina intercourse, but that you just don't find it sexy. OK, start there. There are a million sexual activities in the world, and for each one there are people who think it's hot (even if they've never done it, even if they're only thinking about it) and people who find it about as hot as cold stale porridge. Even "normal" fucking.

So, the first question: Is it all that important to your master that you are aroused by fucking? Is obedience enough, of perhaps you concentrating on the fact that this activity is pleasing and arousing him, and this gives you satisfaction? For many masters, this is enough. Actually, many dominants have a wide range of activities that they like to inflict on the slave, and sooner or later they hit something that the slave doesn't care for much, but will do in order to please them. If you're really slave material, you ought to be getting *some* kind of deeper satisfaction from servicing him, regardless of whether it makes you wet.

On the other hand, your master might be the sort who really prefers the slave to be turned on and wanting the activity in question. When a dominant inevitably hits the situation where they run across an activity that they want and the slave hates, they have a limited number of choices:

1) Not do it; find that somewhere else.

2) Do it anyway, and figure out a way to get off on the fact that they're using this willing person, or perhaps even get off on the fact that they don't like it much. I'm a sadist, so that's not so hard for me; if your master does not have sadism as one of his fetishes, that may not work for him.

3) Try and find ways to eroticize it for them. This will vary in efficacy, depending on how easy you are to shape in that way. I've had good results with some things with my boy, but he's a very malleable person, and the presence of testosterone makes the brain more sexually malleable and programmable. It's harder for girls, and even harder for girls with very little sexual experience. (I'm afraid that the fact you are a virgin is a bit of an issue here. In some ways, estrogen-people who have not had regular sex may take some years to figure out how

their body most wants to have sex, and what works the best. Be patient.)

I suggest first trying porn. Lots of porn with male-female fucking, since it's heterosexual intercourse that you're trying to program yourself to find sexy. In fact, I'd suggest that you try a variety of different straight fucking porn videos while masturbating on your own. It doesn't matter *how* you masturbate at first; the idea is to create a sustained period of arousal while watching this, and thus eroticize the activity. If this works, repeat the activity while inserting a dildo and then masturbating however you do it. Using dildoes in masturbation is a good way to associate the feeling of penetration with sexual arousal, and you can start small and build up over time.

If visual porn doesn't work, you might try word-porn, before jerking off. Or even fantasizing yourself (but the neat thing about porn is that it gives you images to use in fantasies, where you might be a little too vague to get your crotch going otherwise). If absolutely nothing works, then you need to not be guilty over the fact that this activity simply isn't a turn-on for you, and your master is going to have to resort to numbers one or two in the aforementioned list.

If what he's complaining about is that you can't orgasm during intercourse (or can't do it without other stimulation besides just a thrusting penis), well, according to statistics, surprisingly, many women can't. So you're not alone. Some learn to do it, but that depends on how malleable and reroutable your sexual responses are; some people's are really easy to change and some people are impossible to change, it's just hardwired.

If he really loves you, he will try to understand that this is the way you are, once you've plumbed the edges of "this" and figured out what it is, exactly, that you are. But please don't ignore the gorilla in the corner. If the thing that turns you on more than anything else is lesbian porn—well, that's an issue that you need to really deal with. It might be in his best interest to let you do it with some girls, just to find out once and for all what's going on. Better to know than to have everything fall apart later when you can't stand it any more. At least, if you are going into a (possibly monogamous?) heterosexual relationship even though your primary interest is in women, it'll be on the table and both of you will be aware of it, and appreciate your ongoing struggle and sacrifice in order to be his slave.

Q: What about when the dominant wants to inflict pain and the submissive isn't a masochist? Is it healthy for them to submit to pain anyway? Should they dissociate, go away in their head, in order to get through it?

Raven: I expect that whether that might work would depend on the top in question, and whether they would allow that sort of thing. For some, they just want to able to beat someone for their own pleasure, and don't care much how "present" they are. And there's nothing wrong with that; it's one way of doing things. But for myself, I insist that my bottoms be present. If they are dissociating, I do things to force them back, to make them be present. I won't have anyone "going away" when I'm hurting them. If I'm hurting someone, I want them to be all there, to see their reaction in their eyes and their body. If they can't take pain without going somewhere else, then they can find another top.

Of course, this means that sometimes one has to scale back on the pain levels. When I got my boy, he considered himself a heavy masochist. I quickly discovered that this was because he completely dissociated during pain scenes. When I forced him to be present—and forbade him to ever be anything else with me—we discovered that his pain tolerance dropped drastically. Well, it's more important that he be present than that he be a whipping-post. (I have other friends who really *are* heavy masochists, and if I just want to whale on someone, I can play with them.)

So we scaled way back to simple spankings—and that was immensely humiliating for him, having to go back to "baby" painplay and work on his tolerance. We've found that he has much more of a tolerance when he's extremely aroused, which is something that those of you who aren't masochists but have sadistic tops might ask your dominants to do—get the bottom so turned on that they're in the desperate-to-come stage, and then go back and forth between pain and pleasure for a while. This takes some skill on the part of the top, though, and a good knowledge of the bottom's body and responses.

If my primary use for a slave was as an S/M bottom, that would have been a problem. But since I have access to that elsewhere, for me a slave is more about service and submission, and he's excellent at that. So although it still disappoints him that he can't give me that, and we have to do painplay in small light bits, it's OK for now. And we are slowly eroticizing pain, bit by bit.

For those who are not currently slaves but would like to up your pain tolerance for a potential future owner, it is possible to combine small amounts of pain—things that you can set up and remove yourselves, like clamps or spikes or self-flagellation or overly large penetration—with masturbation. It's a matter of conditioning. You start small and light, you work your way up only as quickly as you feel comfortable with. You push yourself a little, but not so much that it becomes un-erotic. It's far better than dissociating. Save that for the nonconsensual pain that Nature doles out.

Joshua: When we first started out, I was very devoted and obedient and I wanted very badly to take these beatings to please my master. I am quite good at getting up a positive attitude for all manner of potentially unpleasant tasks for service to him, so I submitted to them without complaint, and felt 100% that it was right and appropriate for my master to use me in this way.

I don't have childhood abuse issues. My parents never did anything worse than flicking my forehead to get my attention. I've never been struck in anger by a lover. I have never been physically disciplined by anyone in my entire life, or subjected to prolonged physical hardship of any kind. ... but it still screwed me up. Early on, we did a handful of serious no-limits beat-down scenes. After the fact I was proud of having taken them and very turned on by the marks, but the scenes were very hard for me to deal with. I certainly didn't resent my master for doing it, but what our hearts and minds know is sometimes different than what our bodies know.

I remember standing in the kitchen around that time and my master raised his hand to touch my hair. Without any thought, I flinched from him. He has never once made the slightest threat to strike me outside of clearly defined scene or sex play, and I had no reason to think he'd ever backhand me in the kitchen without warning or cause. I flinched anyway. It took about six months for my body to forget about those beatings.

Even though it was emotionally very painful for both of us, he decided to stop beating me entirely. I screamed and begged and gave him all manner of hard time over this, but he had made his decision. He let me have my tantrums, and patted me on the head, and told me this was the way it had to be. It was months before he would even do slightly rough sex. What seemed like ages later, he started gradually incorporating into our sex play the types of pain that I found the most erotic (biting, grabbing, cuttings and bloodplay, very rough fucking), and many months after that he started with occasional light spankings. The process has been incredibly humbling for me.

We're at the point now where on the rare occasion when he decides to spank me (once every month or so) I generally get desperate for him to hurt me more than he's inclined to do with his bare hand, and I try to beg him to use his belt or something. He doesn't. I try politely and respectfully suggesting afterward that I am ready to take more than that. No response.

He'll do this exactly as he sees fit to do this, and he is not particularly interested in my suggestions. He'll listen to me, but he feels that he understands this process a lot better than I do. When I calm down, it is pretty clear to me that he is right, and that no good would come from him taking my suggestions on this matter. But this process of slow eroticization seems to be working; it's just hard for me to accept how slow it has to be in order to work deeply.

Q: Do you use safe words in S/M even in full-time enslavement dynamics?

Joshua: Most heavy M/s folks don't, because the slave consented at the beginning of the relationship to endure anything that their owner wanted, and to trust them on it. In theory, I could use a safeword during play, to get a short reprieve. Two minutes, maybe five. He'd likely check on me, fix any immediate discomfort problems, and let me breathe and get my head back together ... and then he would go back to doing whatever it is that he was doing. I've never used one. Not because I'm oh-so-slavey, but because I'm a "let's get it over with" sort of person. It has been entirely irrelevant for a few years now, but I think it is still "on the books".

I suppose a master might decide that they do not want to force their slave into anything, and give them a safeword (for play or daily life) to make certain of that. Some owners prefer to focus on modifying the slave's will rather than training obedience. Rather than making the slave do things they don't want, they change the slave until they want to do the right things. The owner might find that for this particular slave, a clear line saying "You are doing this by choice. You could stop it at any time," is paradoxically the best way to bring about that modification of will. I can imagine that working well with a slave who was particularly rebellious. The owner gives them nothing to rebel against.

It reminds me of a couple I heard from where the dominant's only response to the submissive's disobedience was to address them by their given name (rather than "slave") and treat them like an equal until they modified their behavior.

Q: What does "subspace" mean?

Joshua: For me, that can mean a lot of different things. Examples:

❖ My master can drop me into a light-to-moderate trance fairly instantly, out of nowhere, especially if we've been working with it frequently. It is sort of a hypnotic conditioning type of thing.

❖ With prolonged sexual arousal just short of orgasm, he can put me in what I call the "fuck me with a tractor" headspace, where all manner of painful things are wonderful and reality goes all squidgy.

❖ I've experienced a clean endorphin high from suturing play, with no D/s component to it. I think it took about 10-15 minutes to get me high out of my mind, and it went on for maybe 30-45 minutes all told. I got there when I was branded, too. Maybe took 5-10 minutes. Those were the only times I'd gotten into a seriously altered state from pain.

❖ I usually get some level of altered awareness when bottoming in any kind of SM scene—the whole universe narrows to this little bubble around me and I have little or no awareness of anything beyond that. Often if the top is making no direct physical contact with me and is using a long whip-type implement, they are outside this "bubble". That is always a little unsettling to me, and it is the reason I tend to prefer wrestling, biting, smacking, kicking and punching to whips and canes and floggers.

The fourth state has much less of a clear physiological response than the other three. It is a matter of degree and comes on gradually, to varying levels of intensity, so it is hard to say how long it takes to get there. In the other three there is a clear moment when things *shift*, as if a flood of brain chemicals is released and suddenly my perception of reality is markedly different. I could time it if I wanted to. They are very clearly either on or off.

Q: Why would you use humiliation in such a delicate relationship? Surely you don't want your slave to be traumatized or have low self-esteem.

Raven: There are two possible ways in which this kind of thing can actually be very positive. (Beyond simply making the various parties hot!)

First, if you talk to long-term experienced submissives who've been with a single dominant for a long time, many of them will talk about how specific activities were once humiliating, but now they're just another way in which they serve. This is a matter of desensitization. Everyone has something that they're embarrassed about, but through careful, deliberate, mindful humiliation "work"—I hesitate to use the word "play", even though it can be couched that way—people can become desensitized to most of the things that embarrass them, until almost nothing can get to them—and that is a good thing.

Second, sometimes people have deep dark secrets that they are ashamed of, usually because they aren't socially acceptable—an example would be a fantasy that can't be done in real life because bad things would happen—and that they fear other people knowing about. Sometimes the emotions regarding these things are a tangled, ambivalent mix of shame and desire, pleasure and anguish. Having a trustworthy person who knows these things about you, doesn't think any the less of you for having this, and (if possible) is willing to go there with you and trigger that mix of emotions, perhaps doing things to enhance the pleasure side, or at least make you feel that you're not too much of a monster for it, can be a very healing experience. It's a way to have that shame have less of a hold on you, and that's always good. But you have to know what buttons you can and can't push. For some people, for example, verbal abuse is a big deal. For some, it's not.

Q: My master wants me to top him. Isn't that inappropriate?

Raven: I haven't got a submissive bone in my body, but sometimes I like pain, or I want to lay back and get done in whatever way I'm fantasizing in my head. And what the heck is a sex slave for if they can't help you act out your selfish fantasies and fetishes, whatever dirty perverted thing they might be?

To me, a slave who says, explicitly or implicitly, "I will only obey you if you act sexually within the confines of a certain narrow role" isn't really a slave, and you don't really own them. They are a "slave", and they are subtly dictating to the "owner" how they think an owner ought to act. They're basically saying, "My slave status is so mentally fragile in my head that if you order me to do anything that isn't in character with my fantasy, I'll slip out of it ... so I'm refusing, probably passive-aggressively, and I'm going to try to push you back toward being the top of my fantasies, so I don't have to struggle with how much of a slave I'm not." This ends up being another form of the "slave" whose "owner" can tell the "slave" to do anything the "slave" wants. I don't like the idea that a slave would put sexual limits on me out of disliking a (nonharmful) activity.

In my view, a good slave should strive to do whatever their owner wants sexually, within physical limits. If an owner expresses interest in being topped, and the slave is at a loss, their response should be, "Master/Mistress, I don't know how to do that properly, but if you train me or have me trained by someone knowledgeable, I would be glad to provide any kind of stimulation that you like."

I've also known female-type subs who are weird about the idea of being ordered to don a strap-on and screw someone. It messes with their gender, and how their gender interacts with their submissiveness, and all sorts of things. Which I think is good for anyone, psychologically. It's good to be stretched once in a while. (I've also run across some slaves who protest loudly that they could never do anything like that, and that their master has no interest in that at all, and in fact would be disturbed to imagine that their slave might even be capable of such things, and one wonders if the loud protest is a way of reassuring their master that they really are the slavey-slave he thinks they are.)

I like to get fucked—sometimes rather roughly—and I like pain on occasion. What I don't like is surprises, and not being in control of the situation implicitly. I will unashamedly top from the bottom in these situations, and I know that no self-respecting dominant is going to put up with the way that I like it. So training a slave to occasionally top me in exactly the way I want is the best way to go.

As far as a sub who's willing but might start thinking, in the middle of the scene, that they're the dominant; well, there are ways to get around that. Like Joshua points out below, you can suddenly stop them in the middle and say, "Never mind. Go make me a sandwich." Make sure to do it after you have your orgasm, but before they get one. As they wander off bewilderedly to the kitchen, it's driven home who's in charge. Also, explicitly topping from the bottom—"More to the left, boy"—helps too.

I know quite a few dominants (and I don't mean switches) who have fantasies about getting topped or dominated, but it's just a sexual fantasy. The truth is that they don't really want to be dominated by someone all the time, or even further than a few hours of play, maybe a weekend. And if you prod further, you find out that what they really want is not to be dominated in reality, but to be dominated exactly the way that they imagine it in their mind—sometimes down to the last detail.

They want their fantasy of submitting, which often has nothing to do with the reality of it. They want the catharsis, or the attention, or they just want to play out a fun fantasy that's been brewing in their heads.

And you know what? There's nothing wrong with that, as long as they're honest about it. And if that's what you want, well, the best partner for it is a service-oriented submissive who can play at being dominant—in exactly the way that the dominant wants—and not actually try to make them do what the "acting top" might prefer. I think that most of the people who pay for domination are like this. People give them shit for not being "really" submissive, and they aren't—many are high-powered executives or people with a lot of responsibility in their lives, and it's OK if they want to give it all up for two hours in a safe space, and then take it back again.

A good slave will easily be able to tell the difference between actually having the upper hand in the relationship, and being told, "OK, I want you to strap this on—this one here!—and then make me suck it, and then beat me—not there, a little to the left—OK, now fuck me till I come. OK, now snuggle me. OK, now go make me dinner." If they are still so fixated on pigeonholing ply activities that they can't see who is really in charge here, then they aren't getting it.

Granted, a slave can only provide the services that they are trained to, and capable of, providing. My boy's worked as a service top from long before he met me, and he is quite good at putting on a convincingly dominant attitude for about an hour, all the while watching the person closely to make sure that he's tailoring the experience entirely to their needs. I've topped other dominants who were friends and needed a good beating for cathartic reasons, and I have no illusions that they would bring me a drink at the next munch. It's discreet, and an act of friendship and respect for someone who has a need to be met quietly on the side.

There are also many sexual acts that I like but would rather not discuss except under very specific and safe circumstances, and I do those with Joshua, who is happy to engage in any sort of perversion that I might cook up, without judging or tattling. I don't suggest them to casual pickups. I'd think that if you had a slave who was a good actor, they could easily be the dominant's top-whore, as it were, and everybody is happy. After all, it's just a service. I am very much in favor of The Owner Gets What They Want Sexually, And The Slave Should Learn To Provide It Happily, No Matter What It Is.

Joshua: I assume that we're not talking about manipulative "topping from the bottom", but a good and obedient submissive or slave providing sexual services of a "toppy" variety. A lot of dominant folks are big ol' pervs with all manner of kinks, and some get hot over being smacked around and fucked once in a while—provided it is exactly the way they like it and they are in complete control.

I'm a slave, but I genuinely enjoy topping, both sexually and in S/M. (I'm a big ol' perv too.) I've "topped" dominant folks a few times and when you get down to it, it's just another sort of sexual service. I'll give a dominant a beating in exactly the way they like it, if that is their kink, and if they get bored and say, "Never mind, go make me a sandwich." then I'll go make them a sandwich. I've known of a few otherwise very good and obedient subs who totally balked at the idea of giving the top a spanking or sexually penetrating them, though.

A former lover and I used to wrestle occasionally, and it would always lead to the "winner" having their way with the "loser". Well, he outweighed my scrawny self by a hundred pounds and was a wrestler all through high school and college, so it is surprising how often I "won". Sometimes control would flip back and forth several times in an evening, and that was a great time. We didn't have a D/s relationship, but still, I'd enjoy it if a dominant I was "topping" decided he'd had enough and took me down, especially if it was sudden and unexpected. I'll happily fight or be passive, whichever they prefer.

My prior experience with BDSM was both topping and bottoming. I'm actually very fond of topping other subs for humiliation scenes, and I enjoy doing "training"-type interactions with subs. I picked up a little skill with flogging and bondage, although I don't find them inherently erotic. But service-oriented submissive folks often make the best professional dominants! It's very much a service to top someone exactly the way they like it, when they choose to ask it of you, regardless of what you might prefer to do with them or whether you'd otherwise be particularly interested in doing anything with them right now. Some professional dominants are much more dominant than that, but frequently it is at heart a professional service of helping the client live out their fantasies.

Q: Do you keep your slave in a cage?

Raven: Er … no. One could, if one was into that sort of thing. Some dominants use a cage as a sort of "time-out" area for their submissives. Others just do it because it gets them off.

Joshua: I don't believe my master has ever put me in long-term bondage. He'll occasionally do a little bondage with his play partners just to make sure the bottom doesn't squirm and wind up getting hit in the face or hands, but only if he is really pushing their pain limits or if they are likely to panic and lash out, or try to get away. Sometimes he likes to tie me up and then fuck me or make me lick his boots, but it's not a big thing for him. Usually he just tells me to hold still, and I do.

I think my master's general stance on confinement is that I am of no use to him in a cage. He doesn't keep me only because he enjoys my submission for its own sake. He keeps me because I am useful and I do as I am told. Any amusement value in caging or confining me would be over the first time he had to get his own drink.

Conclusion

When two people are just trying to explore D/s or M/s relationships, there may be few good models for them to follow, at least that they can find close to home. Since it's not something that you can always talk about to your egalitarian friends, this is often isolating to a couple who are attempting this, and they can find themselves with no one to talk to when they run into problems. Deep power dynamics are not always acceptable in the local kink communities, and even in the smaller M/s-oriented groups, it often seems like you're supposed to know everything already, to have every part of your dynamic greased and smooth and working perfectly, or you'll be shamed in front of those proud owners and polished properties. This can really make it hard for people who need help and don't know where to ask.

Knowing this has made it all the more poignant when people come up to us after a workshop to quietly ask their questions, or email us with these holes (and hopes) in their hearts, or even bravely post their vulnerabilities to a public list. It was a privilege to be allowed to look into the personal lives of other couples (and triples!) working their way toward M/s. May you all find what you desire, and get what you need. May you never be afraid to ask for help, and may you find the spirit inherent in this narrow path.

RAVEN KALDERA AND JOSHUA TENPENNY

Appendix A: Our Contract

(When we started writing this, we found damn few useful models that weren't riddled with fetishy or unrealistic rules. Since then, one of the most common questions that we've been asked is, "What should we put in a contract?" Obviously that's going to be very personal between the people involved, but we're providing ours as an example to inspire people. We wanted something that could adapt to changing and fickle sexual desires, and would outline our expectations of each other ... and most importantly, reassure each other that we were both on the same page. This contract won't talk about "slave positions" and buttplugs and webcams. It does, however, have slightly flourish language ... blame Raven for that. He's just like that.)

Contractual Service Obligations for Raven's Boy Called Joshua Allen Tenpenny, In Service to Raven Kaldera Regis, King of Asphodel

Having held to the former edition of this contract for a year and a day, and having decided with all due deliberation to renew it again for this coming year, Raven Kaldera Regis, King of Asphodel, hereby accepts again Raven's Boy, called Joshua Allen Tenpenny, into his service for an indefinite period of time. During this period of service, Joshua will submit his person and himself to the mastery of his Lord.

With this contract, we enter into a sacred partnership of mastery and submission. Joshua will formally undertake the path of spiritual service to Raven and, through him, to the Gods. Raven will take on the responsibility of gracious acceptance and honorable use of the gift Joshua offers to him; he will strive always to be worthy of Joshua's trust, and to be above malice and pettiness. We both submit ourselves to the Gods for judgment should we fail in our trust.

We agree that the virtues of trust, honesty, openness, loyalty, honor, and integrity will be fundamental to Joshua's service to Raven, and also to Raven's care of Joshua. Joshua will not be required to do anything unethical, dishonorable, or against the edicts of his gods. Should he behave dishonestly or dishonorably, Raven may declare the contract null and void, and choose to release him from this service. In counterpart, should Raven act with repeated and unrepentant dishonor and disregard for Joshua's well-being, Joshua can declare this contract null and void, since he cannot honorably serve a dishonorable master.

Joshua will be an integral part of the Cauldron Farm family, clan, and household. His needs will be taken into consideration at family meetings. He will treat each member of the household with the respect and deference due to their position. He will always have a place in our bed, under our roof, at our table, and in our hearts. Raven will have the following ownership rights over Joshua:

Absolute access to body. Joshua's flesh and blood belongs entirely to Raven, and he may do with it what he wishes. In his turn, Raven will endeavor not to damage his property, and to provide adequate food, shelter, clothing, rest and sleep time, and medical care.

As an extension, Raven also has absolute access to any and all physical property and resources belonging to Joshua, although he may simply request that Joshua steward those resources carefully until such time as Raven chooses to access them.

Raven has the right to demand sexual service from Joshua at any time that he chooses, although as with all tasks, Joshua's physical and mental state will be taken into consideration.

No one else has any access to Joshua's flesh without applying respectfully to Raven for permission, and being interrogated and approved. Raven may deny anyone access to any part of Joshua at any time for any reason, although he agrees to explain the reason to Joshua.

The sole exception to this rule shall be during times of Joshua's service to the Love Goddesses as a sacred prostitute. During these times, he may touch others anywhere, and be touched by them anywhere except between his legs. His genitals will remain off limits and he will not be allowed orgasms with clients. Raven reserves the right to deny him service to any client outside of the Temple of Aphrodite if he so deems them to be a danger to Joshua, the family, the Church, and/or the Kingdom.

Joshua may not exchange bodily fluids with anyone other than Raven and Bella. In return, Raven and Bella both agree to the same restriction, creating a polyfidelitous fluid bond.

Joshua may not ingest any mind-altering substance without permission from Raven. This includes: alcohol, any legal or illegal hallucinogenic, narcotic, or euphoriant plant matter, and any legal or illegal mind-altering pharmaceutical drug.

Joshua shall not intentionally modify his body in any way without Raven's permission. This includes everything from cutting hair to undergoing serious medical treatment.

Absolute access to mind. Joshua has no right to privacy of word, thought, or deed from his master. Raven can demand and expect to get immediate and truthful information on any part of Joshua's life, including dreams, thoughts, fantasies, information, knowledge, and words and deeds past and present. Anything that Joshua knows, thinks, or writes will be at Raven's disposal.

Joshua agrees to learn any specific skills that Raven requires of him, with alacrity and serious application. Raven will be the sole judge of whether a given skill or field of knowledge is beyond his ability, and he will be expected to apply himself repeatedly and persistently over a significant period of time until it is clear to Raven that no further improvement can be made.

Joshua's skills are at Raven's disposal as well. Joshua will make an effort to notice when specific skills of his would be useful, and to volunteer them.

Absolute access to emotions. We agree to a discipline of radical honesty with each other. Neither of us may let resentments pile up without speaking, or lie about how we feel regarding each other or any part of the relationship. We both agree that when asked for our feelings on any matter, they will be open and honest.

Raven may choose to honestly inform Joshua that something is none of his concern. Joshua must reveal his feelings on any matter that interests Raven.

Joshua agrees to maintain an ability to objectively view their relationship, and not allow himself to become a drone, in the best interests of maintaining mental health for both parties.

Raven agrees to take seriously Joshua's feelings and opinions regarding the relationship, Joshua's own mental health, and Raven's behavior towards him. He will never penalize Joshua for being candid with his perceptions, nor require Joshua to baby his ego. However, Joshua also agrees to be reasonably considerate with his negative emotional states, and not take them out on Raven.

Absolute access to will. Joshua agrees to be completely obedient to Raven in any way that Raven commands. He may voice an objection, but he may not refuse any command that does not place him in physical, legal, or ethical jeopardy.

Joshua is not allowed to be submissive in this way to anyone else. He is required to take orders concerning the household management from Bella, and he may play with other tops with Raven's permission and within Raven's presence, but he must conduct himself assertively and independently with everyone else. Full submission is reserved entirely for his master and owner.

The exception to this rule is, of course, submission to the Gods. However, Joshua should refrain from voluntarily making any commitments to the Gods without prior discussion with Raven.

Raven agrees that Joshua shall not be lent to anyone for sexual purposes without Raven being present, and that those purposes will not involve Joshua's genitals, which belong solely to Raven. Although Joshua may not refuse a command to service someone sexually in other ways, he is not required to feign sexual arousal, although he must remain courteous and professional.

Joshua agrees to submit to Raven when his master requires him to suffer pain. He may not refuse to submit, although his physical condition at any given time will be taken into account. A safeword during scenes will allow him time to focus and prepare himself, at his master's discretion, but he has no power to stop any scene or any of Raven's actions during any scene. His suffering is a gift given to his master, and will never be used for purposes of punishment. Joshua agrees to submit with a whole heart, as fully as possible, recognizing the spiritual and emotional necessity of these scenes, and continue to do everything he can to maintain openness toward Raven both during the scene and afterwards.

This relationship will not rely on physical punishment, or restriction of privileges, for discipline. If Joshua fails to correctly obey an order, both the reason for failure and an effective solution will be determined by discussion. For repeated offenses, the master's disappointment and anger, and banishment from the master's presence until further notice, should be punishment enough.

Absolute access to time. Joshua's time and energy are to be scheduled around his usefulness to Raven and to the household. In return, Raven promises to make sure that he has adequate time for rest, sleep, personal care, and following his own hobbies and interests.

Joshua will make himself available for any random personal duty that Raven may require. If he is currently occupied, Raven will make the timetable of that duty clear so that no schedule conflicts occur.

Joshua will endeavor to make the best use of his time, and remain focused on chores that require his immediate attention. If there is a list of chores to be done, Joshua will write them down rather than relying on his memory.

If Raven chooses, he may rent Joshua out to any other person who he deems appropriate to do whatever work they have agreed on. Raven agrees to take Joshua's opinions on the worthiness of the work and the renter into consideration, and not to send him to do work that harms or damages him.

This contract shall stand for one year and one day, at which time it shall be reevaluated, and renegotiated or discarded as we choose.

By our hands this day in May,

Raven Brangwyn Kaldera Regis

Joshua Allen Tenpenny

Appendix 2: Resources

Most of the resources that we list here are not general BDSM resources. Frankly, if you need those, you're not ready for this book, and most are not relevant anyway. These resources fall into two categories: at least part is very useful for the practice of mindful M/s, or else it is useful to servants who want to polish their service. Some we've read ourselves and recommend; others were recommended to us by folks in M/s relationships.

Books:

Dark Moon Rising: Pagan BDSM and the Ordeal Path. Raven Kaldera, 2006. Asphodel Press, Hubbardston MA.

(An entire section on the spirituality of service and mastery. Written by Raven and other very cool people.)

Ask The Man Who Owns Him: The Real Lives of Gay Masters and Slaves. david stein and David Schacter, 2009. Perfectbound Press.

(This book interviews 32 very different gay men who have in common only that they are gay and they are all in Master/slave relationships. Rather than putting out theories, the authors just let the couples (and triples, and more) tell it themselves: their motivations, their protocols or lack thereof, their joys and struggles in these very special relationships. Highly recommended as an array of different real-life models for people to pick and choose from when crafting their own dynamics.)

Where I Am Led: A Service Exploration Workbook. 2nd Edition, 2009. Alfred Press.

(Written by our friend slavette, this is a workbook for submissives and slaves (actual and would-be) who want to learn how to hone their service skills. If you've ever wondered how to give yourself more market value as a sub, start with this book.)

Manual Creation: Defining the Structure of an M/s Household. Machele Kindle, 2007. Nazca Plains Corp.

(Our friend slavette recommends this book, saying: "Very thorough guidance on developing unique master/slave relationship structures. An excellent resource for those who want to create their own household policy and procedure documents.")

To Love, To Obey, To Serve. V. M. Johnson, 1999. Mystic Rose Books.

Slavette also recommends this one, saying: "This is an intimate look at the real life of a slave taken directly from the pages of her journal covering a period from the 1970s to the 1990s. It is part history lesson, part inspiration, and part cautionary tale."

Home Comforts: The Art and Science of Keeping House. Cheryl Mendelson, 2005. Scribner, NYC, NY.

(Joshua's favorite book on housekeeping.)

Miss Manners' Guide to Excruciatingly Correct Behavior, Freshly Updated. Judith Martin, 2005, W.W. Norton and Co.

(Actually, all the Miss Manners books are useful, including the ones on household harmony and communications. It's never a bad thing for a submissive to be unfailingly polite, and frankly it's good for the dominants too. Power dynamics do better with courteous behavioral protocols.)

The Definitive Book of Body Language. Allan and Barbara Pease, 2006. Bantam Press, NY.

(Recommended to us by a domme who uses it to tell when her boy is holding back or having trouble communicating.)

Training Trances: Multi-Level Communication in Therapy and Training. John Overdurf, Julie Silverthorn, and Tad James, 1995. Metamorphous Press.

(Recommended by a lovely Ericksonian/NLP hypnotist-domme friend of ours for beginners who want to work fairly safely with hypnotic techniques.)

While in general we prefer people not to use fiction as the inspiration for real-life relationships, we are cautiously including a few well-written fiction examples here, with the caveat that everyone should recall that they are what they are. That said:

The Marketplace. Laura Antoniou, 2000. Mystic Rose Books.

(This is the first in a series of erotic fiction, and the one that Joshua feels is the most useful of the series, largely as a "morality tale" about submissives and their assumptions and internalized stereotypes, and how they learn to grow beyond those limitations. The book posits a secret "Marketplace" where submissives are trained to be positional-type pure-service slaves and contracted out to rich masters. While it is an engaging read, Raven's issue with the whole series is that there's practically nothing in the way of worthy examples of owners – the trainers pass slaves on and don't keep them, and the owners are rich people who are free to be jerks. That said, Joshua recommends it anyway for the parable involved.)

The Remains of the Day. Kazuo Ishiguro, 1990. Vintage Press.

(Slavette recommends this book and says: "Although completely mainstream, this story explores concepts and ideas that are universal to any service-based relationship. One of the few cases where both the book and the movie are equally good.")

As She's Told. Anneke Jacob, 2008.
Pink Flamingo Publications.

(This is a good fiction example of a couple on the far end of "control-oriented" relationships, from the point of view of both the slave and the master. In spite of how extreme the control gets, we were impressed by the sanity, ethics, and judgment of the master, in a genre full of crazed and unethical tops. Good example of the slow mutual negotiation of a TPE/IE relationship.)

Websites:

The Internet is ever-changing, and one lists websites in a print book at one's peril. They may all be dead by the time you lay hands on this. Still, we'll give it a shot.

Baphomet's Temple: Pagan BDSM
http://www.paganbdsm.org/

(Our website. Lots of stuff on M/s spirituality. Also a place to get our books.)

Broken Toys
http://www.paganbdsm.org/brokentoys/index.html

(Tips to help dominants who have subs with mental illnesses, psychological disorders, and neurological problems.)

Masters And slaves Together – MasT
http://www.mast.net/

(The main national organization for M/s couples, open to anyone who identifies as master/mistress or slave.)

Simply Service.
http://www.submissiveguide.com/ resources/simply-service.

(An online zine for service-oriented submissives. The "mother site" has also been recommended as a useful place for subs to go.)

Internal Enslavement http://www.enslavement.org.uk/

(The original site on internal enslavement. While the authors have some differences with the gender theory prevalent on this site, it's worth reading for the techniques.)

Frugal Domme
http://www.frugaldomme.com

(Recommended to us by some female-dominant/male-submissive couples. While most of it is fetish, there are a few good pages on how to give proper service.)

Master Taino's Resource Site
http://www.mastertaino.com/resources.htm

(This is a pretty comprehensive page for people to look through, including many books, sites, events, clubs, and links to leather families. Master Taino runs the Master/slave conference each year, listed below.)

The Master/slave Conference
http://masterslaveconference.org/

(Official website for the only current conference in America that focuses on D/s/M/s and not just umbrella BDSM stuff. You won't find workshops here on "How To Put A Thousand Needles In One Vagina", but you will find thoughtful and interesting workshops on real-life power dynamic relationships.)

The Master/slave Household Registry
http://www.mshouseholdregistry.com/

(A general listing of many different sorts of M/s households. We include this here, rather than any specific personal M/s household site, as a jumping-off point for people to look at a wide variety of ways to work this.)

About the Authors

By now you ought to know a lot about us, or at least a lot about one major and intimate part of our existence. However, to cover all the things we left out:

Raven Kaldera is a Northern Tradition Neo-Pagan shaman, homesteader, astrologer, herbalist, vampire, and intersexual transgendered FTM activist. He is the King of a very small Pagan kingdom, and one of the founders of its current incarnation, the First Kingdom Church of Asphodel. He is the author of far too many books to list here, but any web search will tell you far more than you want to know.

Joshua Tenpenny is a massage therapist, Asian bodyworker and Shiatsu practitioner who can be found at holisticbodyworking.com. He specializes in helping people get in touch with their bodies for optimum health. (Sorry, all this work is done nonsexually.) He is also a shaman's boy, and considers his service to Raven to be sacred work.

CPSIA information can be obtained at www.ICGtesting.com
Printed in the USA
LVOW07s1128170216

475500LV00001B/40/P